your
wheat
free
gluten-free
DIET PLAN

your *wheat free*

gluten-free
DIET PLAN

carolyn humphries

foulsham
LONDON • NEW YORK • TORONTO • SYDNEY

foulsham

The Publishing House, Bennetts Close,
Cippenham, Slough, Berks, SL1 5AP, England

ISBN 0-572-02672-2

CONTENTS

INTRODUCTION

When you are first told that you have to go on a gluten-free or wheat-free diet, it's devastating. It seems as if just about every basic food is banned. But it really isn't so. True, you can't just grab a sandwich or have any old biscuit with your cup of tea, but with the help of this book, you can create all sorts of gorgeous goodies you thought you'd have to give up. There are golden, light sponge cakes, sumptuous quiches and rich and fruity jam tarts. Crusty bread, chocolate brownies and even sausage rolls are all here. So get cooking and enjoy your new, improved and delicious diet.

If you are sensitive to wheat, you can still include other cereals – such as oats, barley and rye – in your diet. Coeliacs, however, have to avoid all of these as well as wheat. To make this book enjoyable for all, every recipe is completely suitable for both coeliacs and those with wheat sensitivity. For those who can include other cereals in their diet, there is information in the recipe introductions on variations you can try.

Whatever kind of diet you follow, always remember that you need to maintain a good balance of food types. Eat plenty of fresh fruit and vegetables, keep your fat intake to a minimum, avoid too many sugary foods and above all – enjoy!

WHEAT SENSITIVITY

If you are sensitive to wheat, it means you are allergic or intolerant to wheat. It is one of the most common causes of food allergy, but because the symptoms are so diverse, and may also vary greatly in their severity, it is difficult to pinpoint at an early stage. They include muscle stiffness; aching, swollen, red joints; sneezing and watery eyes; stuffed-up or runny nose; migraine; chest pains; nausea; stomach cramps or pains; bloating; skin rashes; swollen throat or trouble in swallowing; sweating; tiredness or apathy; moodiness; irritability or depression; blackouts, panic attacks, flushing, chilling or asthma.

I first came across the condition when my mother was diagnosed with wheat allergy over 20 years ago. She became so poorly that not only was she acutely asthmatic but she was also so debilitated she could only get upstairs on her hands and knees. She was finally rushed into hospital, where, after a multitude of skin tests, blood tests finally confirmed the allergy.

The improvement in her condition when wheat was removed from her diet was phenomenal. And the really big plus is that she has now 'recovered' from the allergy and can take wheat again (although she never overdoes it and avoids wholewheat foods at all costs). Children often grow out of the problem, but many sufferers have to omit wheat from their diet for life.

FOODS TO AVOID IF YOU ARE SENSITIVE TO WHEAT

Below is a list of foods which you should either avoid or be wary of if you are sensitive to wheat. Some brands containing some of the ingredients listed here will be wheat-free, while others will contain wheat in one form or another, so read the labels on everything.

- Baking powder, unless labelled gluten-free – some have wheat flour added as an anti-clumping agent
- Blue cheese – a few specialist cheeses are made using mouldy breadcrumbs rather than chemical moulds

- Bread made with wheat flour – this includes naan, chappatis, pittas, tortillas and rye bread
- Breakfast cereals made with wheat, including muesli
- Bulgar (cracked wheat)
- Cereal binders
- Chinese egg noodles
- Citric acid – some brands are made from wheat
- Couscous
- Dextrins – some may contain wheat and you can't tell
- Durum wheat
- Edible starch – may or may not be made from wheat but you can't tell because the origin of the starch is not stated
- Einkorn wheat
- Farina
- Filler
- Fu (dried wheat gluten)
- Gum base
- Ground spices, especially mixed (apple-pie) spice – may contain wheat flour as an anti-clumping agent
- Hard wheat, including Abyssinian
- Kamut (pasta wheat)
- Miso – may contain wheat
- Modified food starch – may be wheat
- Mono- and diglycerides – may contain wheat
- Mustard powder
- Pasta made with wheat
- Semolina (cream of wheat)
- Shredded (chopped) suet in packets – some brands are coated in wheat flour
- Sodium caseinate
- Soy sauce – some brands contain wheat flour
- Spelt (manna)
- Stock cubes – some brands contain wheat flour
- Triticale
- Udon (wheat noodles)
- Wheat bran
- Wheat flours: plain (all-purpose) flour, self-raising (self-rising) flour, strong (bread) flour, wholemeal flour, granary flour, brown flour, pasta flour, etc.
- Wheatgerm
- Wheat nuts

COELIAC DISEASE

The small intestine is responsible for absorbing all nutrients from our food through the *villi* (fronds) on the intestinal walls. In coeliac disease, gluten (a part of the protein found in wheat, rye and barley) damages the *villi*, literally flattening the fronds so that they cannot absorb the nutrients. Consequently, before diagnosis, coeliacs may suffer from anaemia, osteoporosis, fertility problems (male or female), abdominal discomfort, diarrhoea or unusually short stature. They may also, but much more rarely, show the classic symptoms of tiredness, weight loss and looking wasted and malnourished. Once gluten is removed completely from the diet, the *villi* become restored and function properly again.

Nobody knows how or why it happens, but for all sufferers gluten has to be avoided for life. In babies, the illness produces foul-smelling, pale stools, wind, bloating and poor weight gain and growth. This usually happens soon after cereals are introduced at around six months. It is not advisable for any baby younger than this to have gluten as a small infant's digestive system is too immature to cope with it. If there is any history of coeliac disease in the family, gluten should not be introduced before the baby is one year old.

It was in the late 1800s that the disease was first noticed and it was called chronic intestinal infection (CII). Then, during the Second World War, children in Holland with CII became much better when all the Dutch wheat was exported to Germany. When wheat was available to them again, they became worse. But it was not until 1950 that gluten was identified as the part of the grain that caused the problems.

Dermatitis herpetiformis is a chronic infection of the skin, causing red, sore itchy patches of pustules or blisters. It is often associated with coeliac disease and means a gluten-free diet for life.

FOODS TO AVOID IF YOU ARE COELIAC

There are many conflicting ideas about what can or can't be tolerated by coeliacs, but the information I have given highlights foods to avoid as well as those to be wary of. I have based this on the recommendations of the Coeliac Society. If you have any doubts at all about any foods, check with your gastroenterologist or contact the Society (for their address, see page 187).

- All the wheat products mentioned on pages 7–8
PLUS
- Barley
- Barley malt
- Beer
- Brown table sauce
- Caramel colouring – it may be made from barley
- Lager
- Liquorice sweets – these usually contain wheat flour, although liquorice flavouring is safe
- Malt
- Malt syrup
- Oat bran
- Oatmeal
- Oats
- Oyster sauce
- Pearl barley
- Pure malt extract
- Rice malt
- Rye
- Stout
- Teriyaki sauce
- Tomato ketchup (catsup), some brands – check the label
- Worcestershire sauce

GETTING ROUND THE PROBLEMS

If you are wheat sensitive or coeliac, you cannot eat wheat but you can eat rice in all its forms (and there are masses to choose from these days). You can also choose from wild rice, sago, tapioca, soya, millet, quinoa, amaranth, buckwheat, corn and maize in all its forms, gram flour, urid flour, arrowroot, yam and potato flours. There is also a wheat-free/gluten-free flour available from all good supermarkets. If you are wheat intolerant – but not coeliac – you can also eat oats, barley and rye.

Traditional Italian pasta, which is made from durum wheat, is on the list of forbidden foods, but there are lots of corn, rice and buckwheat pastas available in supermarkets and health food shops, and you can even try your hand at making your own (see page 82).

You can buy commercially made varieties of bread, biscuits (cookies) and cakes in health food shops (at a price!) and a few items, like rice cakes, are available in supermarkets. If you are wheat intolerant you can also eat pumpernickel and whole rye crispbreads. Beware though as many oat, barley or rye products also contain wheat flour. See pages 154–72 for home-baked alternatives.

MYTHS AND FACTS

When you discover that you need to go on a special diet, it is sometimes difficult to sort out the mass of information that may be offered to you – and there are always gaps where you least need them! This list highlights the information that most coeliac and wheat-intolerant people need about common items in their diet.

Alcohol: Coeliacs can drink if they want to. Still and sparkling wines, sherries, ports, vermouths, cider, liqueurs and many spirits, including brandy, gin and rum, are perfectly acceptable but it is recommended that you do not drink beer, stout or lager because these are made from barley. However, there is no evidence that whisky will do you any harm – in moderation of course!

Buckwheat: Buckwheat is not related to wheat in any way and is therefore safe for coeliacs and people with wheat intolerance to eat.

Chips (fries): Home-cooked chips are fine but bought varieties may have an added coating that includes wheat. Chips from your local fish and chip shop may be cooked in oil previously used to cook fish in batter and may cause cross-contamination, so they are best avoided too.

Hydrolised vegetable protein: Coeliacs in America are recommended to avoid this, but there is no evidence, as yet, that it causes problems.

Isomalt: This comes from sugar beet, not barley, and is safe for both coeliacs and people with wheat intolerance. It has a slight laxative effect on some people.

Malt flavouring: This does not cause any problems for wheat intolerance sufferers and the small amount used as a flavour enhancer in cornflakes, for instance, is safe for most coeliacs. If you are think you may be extra-sensitive to it, check with your gastroenterologist. I have avoided the use of any malt in the recipes in this book to make them safe for everyone, but I have used cornflakes. If you are at all unsure, you can buy gluten-free varieties. Coeliacs should avoid all malted drinks and pure malt.

Medicines: Most medication is fine, but some vitamin supplements, for instance, may contain wheat flour or starch as a filler. To be quite certain, check with your pharmacist. Bear in mind that if a medicine upsets your stomach, it is more likely to be caused by the medicine itself than the possibility that it has wheat in it.

Monosodium glutamate: This is a flavour enhancer found in many commercially prepared foods. Although it is made from sugar beet and wheat, after processing, it is unlikely to cause a reaction in both coeliacs and wheat intolerance sufferers.

Oats: Both oats and oat products can be eaten freely by wheat intolerance sufferers, but there is much controversy as to whether or not coeliacs should eat them. Although they do not naturally contain gluten, there is a liklihood of cross-contamination because they are milled in the same factories as wheat. Because of this uncertainty, I have excluded them from this book.

Play dough: Both commercial and home-made varieties are made largely from wheat flour. Unfortunately, bought play dough smells nice and children are often tempted to nibble it, so do make sure coeliac children do not. Recipes for making play dough at home usually contain a huge amount of salt, which should be enough to put children off snacking as they play! Make sure they wash their hands well after use.

Quorn: This is a vegetable protein made from a fungus. The plain minced (ground) kind as well as pieces and steaks are all safe. However, ready-prepared meals made with Quorn, either coated or in sauce, may contain wheat or gluten and so are not suitable.

Soya protein: TVP (textured vegetable protein) is safe, as is tofu (soya bean curd).

Stamps, gummed labels and envelopes: It is a myth that the gum used on these contains gluten so you can safely lick them if you like (personally, I'd rather not anyway!)

Toothpastes, other dental pastes, powders and creams, and mouthwashes: The British Dental Association says all these are safe. The cellulose gum used as a thickener does not contain gluten.

Vinegar: Wine, fruit and cider vinegars are fine. There is some controversy about malt and spirit vinegar. For this reason, I have avoided using them. If in any doubt, check with your gastroenterologist. If you cannot tolerate them, you will need to check the labels of all pickles, dressings and relishes. As an alternative, I have provided some delicious recipes for these items at the end of the book.

READ THE LABELS

Always read the labels and make a note of which brands you discover you can use. For instance, Heinz tomato ketchup (catsup) and baked beans are perfectly suitable but some brands are not. Even baking powder varies – Tesco's own brand is fine but Borwicks contains wheat flour. Where there is doubt, I have called for gluten-free varieties in my recipes. You do not have to go to specialist shops – just check the label before you buy.

A FEW WORDS OF WARNING

- Do not go on any kind of exclusion diet without first consulting your doctor or specialist.
- Some coeliacs are also lactose intolerant. If you are, use non-dairy (i.e. soya) milk, margarine and cream substitutes and the suggested alternatives to cheese in the recipes.
- Although those with wheat intolerance can eat rye, barley and oats, wheat flour is often incorporated with them in commercially produced foods such as rye bread, crispbreads, oatcakes, etc., so do beware.
- Keep checking labels – especially when you notice packaging changes or new claims being made about a product – manufacturers have a nasty habit of changing their formulae from time to time.
- Cross-contamination of even the tiniest quantities can cause problems. At home be scrupulously careful. Breadcrumbs in the butter or jam (conserve), flour left in the pan of your kitchen scales, gluten-free biscuits (cookies) placed in the tin next to ordinary ones could all cause a flare-up of symptoms. Be careful of bought foods too. Macaroons, for instance, are gluten-free but may have been stored next to the cream buns or may be served with the same tongs. A bakery may offer specialist gluten-free products but you cannot be sure they have not been in contact with the rest of the produce. It is also possible for gluten-free flours to be cross-contaminated if they are milled or packaged in close proximity to wheat flour. To minimise the risk, always buy pre-packed varieties made by a reputable manufacturer.

A DIET FOR HEALTH AND WELL-BEING

Every day we all need to have foods in varying quantities from all the five main food groups given below.

Carbohydrates for energy: There are two types of carbohydrates – complex and simple. The complex ones are all the starchy foods like bread, pasta, rice, cereals and potatoes. If you are wheat intolerant, your choice is slightly more limited than usual because ordinary bread, pasta and many breakfast cereals have to be avoided. You should eat plenty of starchy carbohydrate for energy, so look at pages 11–14 for the alternative grains you can have. Simple carbohydrates are sugars. These are found naturally in many foods from fruit to milk, but are also manufactured commercially in many forms, such as all types of granular sugars and syrups, black treacle (molasses) and honey. Plenty of sugar is contained naturally in foods and all the extra you add to biscuits (cookies), cakes and puddings just piles on unnecessary calories. So keep added sugars to a minimum.

Proteins for body growth and repair: Protein is found in lean meat, poultry, game, fish, eggs, dairy products, pulses and manufactured vegetable proteins such as soya protein, tofu (bean curd) and Quorn. If you are also lactose intolerant, avoid dairy products (although you may be able to tolerate hard cheese and yoghurt, goats' and sheep's milk). Eat two or three small portions of protein a day.

Vitamins and minerals for general well-being: The best sources are fruit and vegetables. These should, ideally, be fresh, but varieties that are frozen or canned in water or natural juice are fine too. Eat at least five portions a day.

Fibre for healthy body functioning: Eat plenty of fruit, vegetables, nuts, seeds, dried fruit and skins on potatoes plus the cereals you can eat (see pages 11–14).

Fat for warmth and energy and to protect the skin, muscles and organs: All you need is found naturally in foods, so keep added fat, in the form of butter, margarine or oils, to the minimum, and eat any fat sparingly.

FEEL THE DIFFERENCE IN JUST SEVEN DAYS

Here are some sample menus to get you started. Mix and match as you like but remember, variety is the key and bear in mind colour, texture and flavour when planning meals. I have chosen a different treat and bread for each day, but in reality you would probably use up one batch of baking before starting another.

MONDAY

Breakfast	Glass of pure orange juice Blueberry Quinoa Porridge (page 25) Slice of Crusty White Bread (page 155), butter or margarine and marmalade

Lunch	Sausage Rolls (page 66) with Sweet
	    Chutney (page 185) and tomato and
	    cucumber
	An apple

Teatime treat	Vanilla Fork Cookie (page 163)
Dinner	Chicken Maryland (page 69) Slice of Chocolate Roulade (page 142)

TUESDAY

Breakfast	Half a grapefruit Spiced Hadock Kedgeree (page 32)
Lunch	Potato Pan Pizza (page 60) Plain yoghurt and honey
Teatime treat	Slice of Jam Sponge (page 170)
Dinner	Plum Barbecued Spare Ribs (page 93) Far Eastern Salad (page 133) Peach Almond Crisp (page 143)

WEDNESDAY

Breakfast	Glass of pure orange juice Strawberry Yoghurt Munch (page 27) Slice of Milk Bread toast (page 156), butter or margarine, marmalade
Lunch	Rustic Liver Pâté (page 59) with Sesame Crackers (page 159), side salad A nectarine
Teatime treat	Slice of Moist Fruit Cake (page 172)
Dinner	Traditional Fish 'n' Chips (page 121), Tartare Sauce (page 182) and peas Lemon Sorbet (page 150)

THURSDAY

Breakfast	Glass of pure grapefruit juice Sausages with Tomatoes and Mushrooms (page 30)
Lunch	Broad Bean and Spinach Soup (page 39) A nectarine
Teatime treat	A Rich Chocolate Brownie (page 160)

Dinner	Millet Couscous with Garlic Chicken
	    (page 70)
	Zabaglione with Fresh Pineapple
	    (page 151)

FRIDAY

Breakfast	Slice of melon Honey Nut Crunch (page 23) Plain Breakfast Muffin (page 21), butter or margarine, cherry jam
Lunch	Home-made Burger (page 64) An apple
Teatime treat	No-bake Muesli and Ginger Finger (page 162)
Dinner	Warm Salmon and Citrus Salad (page 98) Slice of Bakewell Tart (page 146)

SATURDAY

Breakfast	Glass of pure orange juice Baked Ham and Eggs with Cherry Tomatoes (page 29) Crusty Bread toast (page 155), butter or margarine and marmalade
Lunch	Spring Vegetable and Bean Soup (page 43) A banana
Teatime treat	A Florentine (page 165)
Dinner	Buckwheat Lasagne al Forno (page 82), a green salad Pear and Yoghurt Brûlée (page 145)

SUNDAY

Breakfast	Slice of melon American-style Buckwheat Pancakes (page 22) with bacon and maple syrup
Lunch	Asparagus Omelette (page 65) Fromage frais with raisins
Teatime treat	Slice of Banana Bread (page 158)
Dinner	Honey Roast Ham in Cider (page 94) with Mustard Seed Potatoes (page 124) and Cauliflower and Broccoli Cheese (page 123) Apple Crumble (page 135)

NOTES ON THE RECIPES

- All ingredients are given in imperial, metric and American measures. Follow one set only in a recipe. American terms are given in brackets.

- All spoon measures are level: 1 tsp = 5 ml;
  1 tbsp = 15 ml

- Eggs are medium unless otherwise stated.

- I have called for gluten-free ingredients where there is any doubt as to the suitability of some brands, so please check the labels.

- I have given the choice of butter or margarine in the recipes. Use a dairy-free alternative if you are lactose intolerant and check it is suitable for cooking, not just for spreading. You will also need to use non-dairy (i.e. soya) milk, cheese and cream.

- Always wash, peel, core and seed, if necessary, fresh produce before use.

- Seasoning and the use of strongly flavoured ingredients such as garlic or chillies is very much a matter of personal taste. Adjust seasonings to suit your own palate and digestion.

- Always use fresh herbs unless dried are specifically called for. If you wish to substitute dried for fresh, use only half the quantity or less as they are very pungent. Frozen, chopped varieties have a better flavour than the dried ones.

- All can sizes are approximate as they vary from brand to brand. For example, if I call for a 400 g/14 oz/large can of tomatoes and yours is a 397 g can, that's fine.

- Cooking times are approximate and should be used as a guide only. Always check that food is thoroughly cooked through before serving.

BREAKFASTS

Breakfast is a very important meal but is the one that you may find the most tricky to deal with. Many ordinary breakfast cereals are full of wheat and even those that aren't tend to have malt extract in them. This may be a problem for some coeliacs but most sufferers can have ordinary cornflakes or puffed rice. Those of you with wheat intolerance can have these and porridge oats or oatmeal too. Ordinary breads, toast, rolls, etc. are no-nos, so try any of my bread, biscuit (cookie) and cake recipes on pages 155–72. For more ideas, have a look at the recipes in this section – any of them will make you a delicious breakfast to set you up for the day. Try to have a small glass of pure fruit juice or some fresh fruit with your meal, to help absorb any iron in the grains and to give you added vitamin C.

Plain Breakfast Muffins

These are also good split and buttered for tea. For a delicious variation, add 30 ml/2 tbsp raisins and 2.5 ml/½ tsp ground cinnamon to the mixture.

MAKES 8

Sunflower oil, for greasing

100 g/4 oz/1 cup wheat-free/gluten-free flour

A pinch of salt

5 ml/1 tsp gluten-free baking powder

20 g/¾ oz/1½ tbsp butter or margarine, softened

15 ml/1 tbsp caster (superfine) sugar

200 ml/7 fl oz/scant 1 cup milk

---

1 Grease eight sections of a tartlet tin (patty pan) with oil.

2 Sift the flour, salt and baking powder together in a bowl.

3 Add the butter or margarine and work in with a fork until the mixture resembles breadcrumbs. Stir in the sugar.

4 Mix with the milk and beat to form a smooth batter.

5 Pour into the prepared sections of the tin and bake in a preheated oven at 200°C/400°F/gas mark 6 for 10 minutes until risen and golden and the centres spring back when lightly pressed. Transfer to a wire rack. Serve warm or cold.

American-style Buckwheat Pancakes

175 g/6 oz/1½ cups buckwheat flour

10 ml/2 tsp gluten-free baking powder

A good pinch of salt

30 ml/2 tbsp caster (superfine) sugar

2 eggs, beaten

300 ml/½ pt/1¼ cups milk

Sunflower oil, for frying (sautéing)

Grilled (broiled) bacon (optional) and maple syrup, to serve

1 Mix the flour, baking powder, salt and sugar in a bowl. Make a well in the centre.

2 Add the eggs and half the milk and beat to form a smooth batter. Beat in the remaining milk.

3 Heat a little oil in a frying pan (skillet). Add 30 ml/ 2 tbsp of the batter and cook until risen and golden underneath. Flip over and cook the other side until golden. Slide out on to a plate and keep warm while cooking the remainder.

4 Serve hot with grilled bacon, if liked, and maple syrup.

Honey Nut Crunch

Those on a wheat-free diet can try using rolled oats instead of half or all of the millet.

SERVES 6–8

175 g/6 oz /1½ cups millet flakes

90 ml/6 tbsp chopped mixed nuts

60 ml/4 tbsp clear honey

Milk, to serve

1 Put the millet and nuts in a heavy-based frying pan (skillet) over a moderate heat.

2 Cook, tossing all the time, for a few minutes until golden brown. Do not allow to burn. Turn the heat down to low.

3 Add the honey and stir until well coated. Cook for about 30 seconds until you can smell the sugar but the mixture is not getting over-brown.

4 Tip on to a sheet of non-stick baking parchment and leave to cool.

5 Store in an airtight container. Serve with milk.

Quinoa Porridge

SERVES 1

---

25 g/1 oz/¼ cup quinoa

200 ml/7 fl oz/scant 1 cup water or milk

A pinch of salt

Milk, cream or yoghurt and sugar or honey, to serve

---

1 Wash the quinoa thoroughly in a sieve (strainer). Drain and tip into a non-stick saucepan.

2 Add the water or milk and a pinch of salt.

3 Bring to the boil, reduce the heat and simmer gently for about 20 minutes until soft and moist.

4 Tip into a bowl and serve with a little milk, cream or yoghurt and sugar or honey, to taste.

Blueberry Quinoa Porridge

25 g/1 oz/¼ cup quinoa

15 ml/1 tbsp dried blueberries

5 ml/1 tsp finely grated orange rind (optional)

200 ml/7 fl oz/scant 1 cup water

Clear honey, to taste

Milk, cream or yoghurt, to serve

1 Rinse the quinoa thoroughly in a sieve (strainer).

2 Tip into a non-stick saucepan and add the blueberries, orange rind (if using) and water.

3 Bring to the boil, reduce the heat and simmer gently for about 20 minutes until the grains are soft and moist and most of the liquid has been absorbed.

4 Sweeten to taste with honey. Serve in a bowl with a little milk, cream or yoghurt.

Apricot and Almond Quinoa

25 g/1 oz/¼ cup quinoa

4 ready-to-eat dried apricots, roughly chopped

200 ml/7 fl oz/scant 1 cup milk or water

15 ml/1 tbsp flaked (slivered) almonds

Clear honey, to taste

Milk, cream or yoghurt, to serve

1 Rinse the quinoa thoroughly in a sieve (strainer).

2 Drain and tip into a non-stick saucepan.

3 Add the apricots and milk or water. Bring to the boil, reduce the heat and simmer for about 20 minutes until the grains are soft and moist and most of the liquid has been absorbed.

4 Stir in the nuts and sweeten to taste with honey. Serve in a bowl with a little milk, cream or yoghurt.

Spiced Muesli

Wheat intolerance sufferers can substitute oats for the millet for a change.

SERVES 1

30 ml/2 tbsp millet flakes

1 small handful of cornflakes

15 ml/1 tbsp dried mixed fruit (fruit cake mix)

15 ml/1 tbsp sunflower seeds

2.5 ml/½ tsp ground cinnamon

5 ml/1 tsp light brown sugar or clear honey, or to taste

Milk or yoghurt, to serve

Mix all the ingredients together in a bowl. Add milk or yoghurt and serve.

Strawberry Yoghurt Munch

SERVES 1

25 g/1 oz/½ cup cornflakes

4 strawberries, thinly sliced

1 small carton of thick plain yoghurt

15 ml/1 tbsp clear honey

1 Put half the cornflakes in a bowl or sundae glass.

2 Add half the strawberries in a layer, then half the yoghurt.

3 Repeat the layers and top with a layer of honey. Eat straight away.

Banana Walnut Whip

SERVES 1

1 large ripe banana

1 small carton of plain fromage frais

A little clear honey

15 ml/1 tbsp chopped walnuts

½ quantity of Cinnamon Toast (see page 37), to serve

1 Mash the banana and beat in the fromage frais.

2 Sweeten with honey to taste and fold in the nuts. Spoon into a small bowl.

3 Serve with Cinnamon Toast.

Tropical Smoothie

SERVES 1

1 ripe banana, cut into chunks

1 small ripe mango, peeled and all the flesh cut off the stone (pit)

100 ml/3½ fl oz/6½ tbsp milk

1 small carton of vanilla yoghurt

15 ml/1 tbsp ground almonds

1 Purée the banana and mango with a little of the milk in a blender or food processor until smooth.

2 Add the remaining ingredients and blend again until thick and frothy. Pour into a large glass and serve.

Baked Ham and Eggs with Cherry Tomatoes

SERVES 4

50 g/2 oz/¼ cup butter or margarine

4 slices of lean ham

8 eggs

12 cherry tomatoes, halved

Salt and freshly ground black pepper

1 Divide the butter or margarine between four individual shallow, ovenproof dishes. Place in a preheated oven at 180°C/350°F/gas mark 4 until melted and sizzling.

2 Remove from the oven and lay a slice of ham in each dish. Break 2 eggs into each one.

3 Arrange the halved cherry tomatoes around the edges and sprinkle with salt and lots of freshly ground pepper.

4 Bake for 10–15 minutes until the eggs are cooked to your liking. Serve hot.

Sausages with Tomatoes and Mushrooms

Buy bacon pieces or economy cooking bacon to make the sausages, they're much cheaper and you get a good mix of smoked and unsmoked bacon. You can make the sausages in advance and store in the fridge or freeze them to cook when you are ready.

SERVES 4

---

450 g/1 lb belly pork slices

225 g/8 oz/2 cups bacon pieces

5 ml/1 tsp dried mixed herbs

A little salt and lots of freshly ground black pepper

15 g/½ oz/1 tbsp butter or margarine

15 ml/1 tbsp sunflower oil

100 g/4 oz button mushrooms, sliced

4 tomatoes, sliced

15 ml/1 tbsp chopped fresh parsley

Buttered toast, made with gluten-free/wheat-free bread (buy ready-made or see pages 155–7), to serve

---

1 Cut the rind off the belly pork slices and remove any bones. Cut the meat into chunks.

2 Discard any bones, gristle or rind from the bacon. Cut into small pieces, if necessary.

3 Drop a piece at a time into a food processor with the machine running until finely chopped, or pass through a mincer (grinder).

4 Season with the herbs, salt and pepper.

5 Draw the mixture together into a ball. Remove any odd white stringy bits of gristly pork fat that haven't been chopped.

6 Shape the mixture into small sausages or balls.

7 Grill (broil) on foil on the grill (broiler) rack or dry-fry in a non-stick frying pan (skillet) for about 5–6 minutes, turning occasionally until golden and cooked through.

8 Meanwhile, heat the butter or margarine and oil together in another pan. Add the mushrooms and tomatoes and cook, stirring occasionally, until tender and cooked through. Season with a little salt and pepper and sprinkle with parsley.

9 Serve the sausages with the mushrooms and tomatoes and buttered toast.

Spiced Haddock Kedgeree

If you are lactose intolerant, omit the cream.

SERVES 4

---

350 g/12 oz undyed smoked haddock fillet, skinned

50 g/2 oz/¼ cup butter or margarine

2 spring onions (scallions), chopped

100 g/4 oz button mushrooms, sliced

225 g/8 oz/1 cup long-grain rice, rinsed and drained

1.5 ml/¼ tsp cayenne

Salt and freshly ground black pepper

10 ml/2 tsp lemon juice

300 ml/½ pt/1¼ cups water

2.5 ml/½ tsp garam masala

4 eggs

20 ml/4 tsp single (light) cream

30 ml/2 tbsp chopped fresh parsley or coriander (cilantro), to garnish

---

1 Cut the fish into bite-sized chunks, discarding any bones.

2 Heat the butter or margarine in a large frying pan (skillet). Add the spring onions and mushrooms and fry (sauté) for 2 minutes, stirring.

3 Add the rice, cayenne, some salt and pepper and the lemon juice, stirring until every grain of rice is glistening.

4 Add the fish and water. Bring to the boil, reduce the heat, cover and simmer very gently for 20 minutes until the rice is cooked and has absorbed nearly all the liquid. Stir in the garam masala. Taste and add a little more salt and pepper, if necessary.

5 Make four 'wells' in the mixture and break an egg into
each. Spoon the cream over each egg. Re-cover and
cook gently for about 10 minutes until the eggs are set.
Sprinkle with parsley or coriander and serve straight
from the pan.

Kippers and Scrambled Egg

You can also make scrambled eggs in the microwave.
Simply whisk the milk and eggs together. Add the butter or
margarine and a little seasoning and cook on High for about
45 seconds per egg, stirring every minute until lightly
scrambled but still slightly 'wet'. Leave to stand for 2 minutes
to complete cooking.

SERVES 4

---

4 boneless kipper fillets

15 g/½ oz/1 tbsp butter or margarine

45 ml/3 tbsp milk

6 eggs

Salt and freshly ground black pepper

**Wheat-free/gluten-free bread (buy ready-made or see
pages 155–7) and butter, to serve**

---

1 Put the kipper fillets in a pan of gently simmering
water. Cover and cook for 5 minutes. Remove with a
fish slice, drain well and transfer to warm plates.

2 Meanwhile, melt the butter or margarine in a non-stick
saucepan. Whisk in the eggs, milk and a little salt and
pepper. Cook over a gentle heat, stirring until
scrambled. Do not allow to boil.

3 Spoon on to the plates with the kippers and serve with
wheat-free/gluten-free bread and butter.

Hash Browns with Crispy Bacon

SERVES 4

4 large floury potatoes, diced

1 large onion, finely chopped

25 g/1 oz/2 tbsp butter or margarine

15 ml/1 tbsp sunflower oil

5 ml/1 tsp paprika

Salt and freshly ground black pepper

4 or 8 rashers (slices) of lean back bacon, rinded

1 Boil the potatoes in lightly salted water for about 5 minutes until just tender. Drain.

2 Meanwhile, fry (sauté) the onion in the butter or margarine and oil in a large frying pan (skillet) for 2 minutes until softened.

3 Add the potatoes, paprika and some salt and pepper. Fry, tossing and pressing with a fish slice, until the potatoes are breaking up and turning golden.

4 Grill (broil) or fry the bacon until crisp and golden on both sides. Serve with the Hash Browns.

The Great English Breakfast

SERVES 4

4 large flat mushrooms

75 ml/5 tbsp water

Salt and freshly ground black pepper

60 ml/4 tbsp sunflower oil

2 cooked potatoes, sliced

4 or 8 rashers (slices) of lean back bacon, rinded

2 large tomatoes, halved

4 eggs

1 Peel the mushrooms if necessary and put them into a frying pan (skillet). Add the water and some salt and pepper. Cover with a lid or foil and cook gently until tender and the liquid has evaporated.

2 Meanwhile, heat half the oil in a second frying pan and fry (sauté) the potatoes until golden on both sides. Transfer to a plate and keep warm.

3 Grill (broil) the bacon and tomatoes, turning once, until the bacon is golden and sizzling on each side and the tomatoes are just tender but still hold their shape.

4 Wipe out the frying pan the potatoes were in and heat the remaining oil in the cleaned pan. Crack the eggs one at a time into a cup, then slide into the pan and fry them until cooked to your liking. Transfer to warm plates.

5 Add the potatoes, mushrooms, bacon and tomatoes and serve.

Bacon and Banana Kebabs on Potato Slabs

Try this too with dried apricots, prunes or mushrooms in the bacon – all are really delicious.

SERVES 4

---

1 very large potato, scrubbed

30 ml/2 tbsp sunflower oil

8 lean rashers (slices) of streaky bacon

4 bananas, each cut into 4 chunks

---

1 Cut the potato lengthways into four thick slices.

2 Heat the oil in a frying pan (skillet) and fry (sauté) the potato slices until golden brown on each side. Cover the pan with a lid, turn down the heat and continue to cook until the slices are tender – about 8 minutes in all.

3 Meanwhile, cut each slice of bacon in half and roll each half round a chunk of banana. Thread on four kebab skewers. Place under a hot grill (broiler) and cook, turning occasionally, until the bacon is golden and the banana is softening.

4 Put the slices of potato on four warm plates. Slide a kebab off the skewer on to each slice and serve hot.

Cinnamon Toast

If making this for one, use half the egg. The other half may be stored in the fridge for later use. For example, to make a sandwich filling for one, beat it with a dash of milk, season and fry (sauté) in a little butter or margarine in a frying pan (skillet). Alternatively, use it for glazing pastry (paste).

SERVES2

1 small egg

30 ml/2 tbsp milk

4 slices of wheat-free/gluten-free bread (buy ready-made or see pages 155–7)

25 g/1 oz/2 tbsp butter or margarine

20 g/¾ oz/1½ tbsp caster (superfine) sugar

5 ml/1 tsp ground cinnamon

1 Beat the egg and milk together. Dip in the bread to coat completely.

2 Fry in the butter or margarine until golden brown on both sides.

3 Mix the sugar and cinnamon together and sprinkle all over the toast. Cut into halves and serve.

SOUPS, STARTERS AND SNACKS

This selection of dishes offers ideal recipes that are light enough to present on their own as starters to whet the appetite. As a bonus, however, most can be combined with one of my tasty breads (see pages 155–7) to make a quick snack, lunch or supper.

Broad Bean and Spinach Soup

SERVES 6

1 onion, finely chopped

15 g/½ oz/1 tbsp butter or margarine

225 g/8 oz shelled fresh or frozen broad (fava) beans

450 g/1 lb fresh or frozen spinach, chopped

900 ml/1½ pts/3¾ cups gluten-free vegetable stock

Salt and freshly ground black pepper

A good pinch of grated nutmeg

15 ml/1 tbsp snipped fresh chives, to garnish

1 Fry (sauté) the onion in the butter or margarine, stirring, for 3 minutes.

2 Add the beans, spinach and stock.

3 Bring to the boil, reduce the heat and simmer gently for 20 minutes.

4 Purée in a blender or food processor and return to the saucepan. Season with salt and pepper and add the grated nutmeg. Reheat.

5 Ladle into warm bowls and sprinkle with snipped chives, to garnish.

Smooth Lettuce and Parsley Soup

This is delicious hot or cold.

SERVES 6

---

1 bunch of spring onions (scallions), chopped

20 g/¾ oz/1½ tbsp butter or margarine

45 ml/3 tbsp cornflour (cornstarch)

600 ml/1 pt/2½ cups gluten-free vegetable stock

1 round lettuce, shredded

50 g/2 oz fresh parsley, chopped

150 ml/¼ pt/⅔ cup milk

60 ml/4 tbsp single (light) cream

Salt and freshly ground black pepper

1 Fry (sauté) the spring onions in the butter or margarine for 2 minutes, stirring, until softened but not browned.

2 Add the cornflour, then remove from the heat and blend in the stock. Return to the heat and bring to the boil, stirring.

3 Add the lettuce and all but 30 ml/2 tbsp of the parsley and simmer for 15 minutes.

4 Purée in a blender or food processor and return to the pan. Stir in the milk and half the cream and season to taste.

5 Either reheat and serve hot, or cool, then chill before serving in soup bowls, garnished with the remaining cream and chopped parsley.

Pea and Carrot Soup with Fresh Mint

SERVES 6

225 g/8 oz shelled fresh or frozen peas

2 large carrots, chopped

900 ml/1½ pts/3¾ cups gluten-free vegetable stock

10 ml/2 tsp caster (superfine) sugar, plus extra for dusting

1 large and 6 small sprigs of mint

Salt and freshly ground black pepper

1 egg, separated

30 ml/2 tbsp single (light) cream

1 Put the peas, carrots and stock in a saucepan with the measured sugar and the large sprig of mint. Add a little salt and pepper.

2 Bring to the boil, reduce the heat, part-cover and simmer for 15 minutes or until the vegetables are really tender. Discard the mint.

3 Purée in a blender or food processor and return to the pan.

4 Meanwhile, brush the small sprigs of mint with the egg white and sprinkle liberally with caster sugar. Place on a sheet of greaseproof (waxed) paper to dry.

5 Whisk the egg yolk and cream together and stir into the soup. Heat through gently, stirring, but do not boil. Taste and re-season, if necessary.

6 Ladle into bowls and serve hot, garnished on the side with a frosted sprig of mint.

Greek Egg and Lemon Soup

You can use raw or cooked bones for this recipe.

1 chicken carcass or lamb leg or shoulder bone

1 litre/1¾ pts/4¼ cups water

1 onion, quartered

1 bay leaf

Salt and freshly ground black pepper

50 g/2 oz/¼ cup long-grain rice

2 eggs

Juice of 1 small lemon

30 ml/2 tbsp chopped fresh parsley, to garnish

1 Break up the carcass, if using, and put the bone(s) in a large saucepan. Add the water, onion, bay leaf and a little salt and pepper.

2 Bring to the boil, skim the surface, reduce the heat, cover and simmer gently for 1½ hours. Strain the stock and return to the rinsed-out saucepan and bring back to the boil. Add the rice and simmer for 10 minutes until tender.

3 Whisk the eggs in a bowl with the lemon juice and 15 ml/1 tbsp water.

4 Add a ladleful of the hot stock and whisk again. Whisk in a second ladleful of stock, then remove the soup from the heat and pour the egg mixture back into the pan. Stir, taste and re-season, if necessary.

5 Ladle into warm bowls, sprinkle with chopped parsley and serve.

Spring Vegetable and Bean Soup

If you are lactose intolerant, omit the cheese if necessary.

SERVES 6

---

1 bunch of spring onions (scallions), chopped

2 carrots, finely diced

1 red (bell) pepper, finely chopped

20 g/¾ oz/1½ tbsp butter or margarine

900 ml/1½ pts/3¾ cups gluten-free vegetable stock

1 bouquet garni sachet

100 g/4 oz spring (collard) greens, finely shredded

425 g/15 oz/1 large can of flageolet beans, drained

Salt and freshly ground black pepper

Grated Cheddar or Parmesan cheese, to serve (optional)

---

1 Fry (sauté) the onions, carrots and pepper in the butter or margarine, stirring, for 3 minutes.

2 Add the stock and bouquet garni sachet and simmer for 20 minutes.

3 Add the greens and beans and simmer for a further 10 minutes. Discard the bouquet garni sachet and season to taste.

4 Ladle into warm bowls and serve with cheese, if liked.

Mediterranean Fish Chowder

SERVES 6

45 ml/3 tbsp olive oil

1 red onion, finely chopped

1 leek, thinly sliced

1 garlic clove, crushed

4 ripe tomatoes, skinned and chopped

1 bay leaf

1 carrot, diced

2 potatoes, diced

1.2 litres/2 pts/5 cups gluten-free vegetable stock

15 ml/1 tbsp tomato purée (paste)

450 g/1 lb white fish fillet, skinned and cubed

100 g/4 oz queen scallops

100 g/4 oz cooked peeled prawns (shrimp)

50 g/2 oz stoned (pitted) black olives, sliced

Salt and freshly ground black pepper

30 ml/2 tbsp chopped fresh parsley, to garnish

1 Heat the oil in a large saucepan. Add the onion, leek and garlic and cook gently, stirring, for 3 minutes until softened but not browned.

2 Add the tomatoes, bay leaf, carrot, potatoes, stock and tomato purée. Bring to the boil, cover, reduce the heat and simmer for 15 minutes.

3 Add the fish and scallops and simmer for 5 minutes. Stir in the prawns and olives and season to taste.

4 Discard the bay leaf. Ladle into warm bowls and sprinkle with chopped parsley before serving.

Easy Tomato, Carrot and Orange Soup

SERVES 4

275 g/10 oz/1 small can of carrots, drained

400 g/14 oz/1 large can of tomatoes

150 ml/¼ pt/⅔ cup pure orange juice

5 ml/1 tsp dried basil

Salt and freshly ground black pepper

20 ml/4 tsp plain yoghurt

1 Put the carrots and tomatoes in a blender or food processor and blend until smooth.

2 Add the orange juice, basil and some salt and pepper and blend again.

3 Heat in a saucepan or chill, then serve in soup bowls with a spoonful of yoghurt on top of each.

Thick Red Lentil and Tomato Soup

SERVES 4

1 large onion, chopped

1 large potato, chopped

1 carrot, chopped

15 g/½ oz/1 tbsp butter or margarine

175 g/6 oz/1 cup red lentils

750 ml/1¼ pts/3 cups gluten-free vegetable stock

400 g/14 oz/1 large can of tomatoes

1 bay leaf

Salt and freshly ground black pepper

30 ml/2 tbsp chopped fresh parsley, to garnish

1 Fry (sauté) the onion, potato and carrot in the butter or margarine, stirring, for 2 minutes until slightly softened but not browned.

2 Add the remaining ingredients and bring to the boil. Part-cover, reduce the heat and simmer gently for 30 minutes until everything is really tender. Discard the bay leaf.

3 Purée in a blender or food processor and return to the pan. Taste and re-season if necessary. Serve hot, sprinkled with chopped parsley.

Bortsch

Do not use beetroot pickled in vinegar for this recipe.

SERVES 4–6

---

2 celery sticks, grated, discarding any strings

1 large carrot, grated

1 onion, grated

3 cooked beetroot (red beets), grated

900 ml/1½ pts/3¾ cups gluten-free vegetable stock

15 ml/1 tbsp cider vinegar

Salt and freshly ground black pepper

20–30 ml/1½–2 tbsp plain yoghurt and 15 ml/1 tbsp snipped fresh chives, to garnish

---

1 Put all the ingredients in a saucepan and bring to the boil. Part-cover and simmer for 20 minutes until everything is soft.

2 Season to taste, ladle into warm bowls and top each with a spoonful of yoghurt and a sprinkling of chives.

Chinese Chicken and Sweetcorn Soup

SERVES 4

100 g/4 oz/1 cup cooked chicken, diced

900 ml/1½ pts/3¾ cups gluten-free chicken stock

5 ml/1 tsp grated fresh root ginger

200 g/7 oz/1 small can of sweetcorn (corn)

15 ml/1 tbsp gluten-free soy sauce

25 ml/1½ tbsp cornflour (cornstarch)

30 ml/2 tbsp dry sherry

Salt and freshly ground black pepper

30 ml/2 tbsp snipped fresh chives, to garnish

1 Put all the ingredients except the cornflour, sherry, salt and pepper in a saucepan. Bring to the boil, part-cover and simmer for 2 minutes.

2 Blend the cornflour with the sherry and stir in. Bring to the boil and cook, stirring, for 1 minute until thickened.

3 Season to taste and serve, sprinkled with snipped chives.

Chicken and Walnut Stuffed Pears, with Creamy Tarragon Dressing

If you are lactose-intolerant, you can use soya yoghurt instead of crème fraîche.

SERVES 6

6 ripe pears

75 g/3 oz/¾ cup cooked chicken, finely chopped

50 g/2 oz/½ cup walnuts, finely chopped

Salt and freshly ground black pepper

150 ml/¼ pt/⅔ cup crème fraîche

Lettuce leaves

30 ml/2 tbsp sunflower oil

10 ml/2 tsp lemon juice

30 ml/2 tbsp chopped fresh tarragon

5 ml/1 tsp caster (superfine) sugar

12 walnut halves and a little paprika, to garnish

1 Peel, halve and core the pears.

2 Mix the finely chopped chicken and walnuts with 15–30 ml of the crème fraîche to bind and season to taste. Spoon into the pear cavities and arrange each one, rounded side up, on a plate of lettuce leaves.

3 Blend the remaining crème fraîche with the oil, lemon juice, tarragon, sugar and a little salt and pepper. Spoon over the pears.

4 Garnish with the walnut halves and a sprinkling of paprika and serve.

Italian Salad with Basil and Olives

If you are lactose intolerant, you may or may not be able to tolerate Mozzarella cheese made with buffalo milk. Check with your doctor or specialist. If not, use thinly sliced firm tofu instead.

SERVES 4

---

4 beefsteak tomatoes, each cut into 6 slices

4 hard-boiled (hard-cooked) eggs, sliced

2 × 125 g/5 oz buffalo Mozzarella cheeses, each cut into 6 slices

12 black olives, stoned (pitted)

8 fresh basil leaves, torn

30 ml/2 tbsp olive oil

15 ml/1 tbsp red wine vinegar

Freshly ground black pepper

1 Arrange the slices of tomato, egg and cheese overlapping each other attractively on four plates. Scatter the olives and basil over.

2 Drizzle the oil and vinegar over the salads and sprinkle with pepper and serve.

Blinis with Smoked Salmon

You can use soya yoghurt instead of soured (dairy sour) cream or crème fraîche if you are also lactose intolerant.

SERVES 4–6

---

1 quantity of American-style Buckwheat Pancake mix (see page 22), omitting the sugar

100 g/4 oz/1 cup smoked salmon pieces

2 onions, finely chopped

150 ml/¼ pt/⅔ cup soured (dairy sour) cream or crème fraîche

Sprigs of parsley and lemon wedges, to garnish

---

1 Make up the pancakes using only 15 ml/1 tbsp of the batter for each one. It should make 16–18 altogether.

2 Arrange on plates with small piles of smoked salmon and onion and a good spoonful of soured cream or crème fraîche to the side of each.

3 Garnish with sprigs of parsley and lemon wedges and serve.

Melon and Cashew Nut Cups

½ cucumber

Salt

6 tomatoes

2 ripe ogen or chanterais melons

50 g/2 oz/½ cup unsalted cashew nuts

15 ml/1 tbsp snipped fresh chives

15 ml/1 tbsp chopped fresh mint

15 ml/1 tbsp caster (superfine) sugar

45 ml/3 tbsp lemon juice

90 ml/6 tbsp olive oil

Freshly ground black pepper

Sprigs of mint, to garnish

1 Peel and dice the cucumber. Place in a colander, sprinkle with salt and leave to stand for 30 minutes. Rinse with cold water and pat dry on kitchen paper (paper towels).

2 Plunge the tomatoes in boiling water for 30 seconds. Drain, remove the skins, halve, discard the seeds and chop the flesh. Place in a large bowl.

3 Cut the melons into halves, remove the seeds and scoop out the flesh using a melon baller or cut it out, then dice. Add to the tomatoes with the cucumber and cashews. Put the melon shells in bowls.

4 Whisk the remaining ingredients together and pour over the melon mixture. Toss gently.

5 Spoon into the melon shells and chill until ready to serve, garnished with sprigs of mint.

Goats' Cheese Medallions with Cranberry Dressing

If you are lactose intolerant, you will need to check if you can eat goats' cheese. Firm tofu would make a good alternative.

SERVES 6

---

3 × 85 g/ 3½ oz cylindrical goats' cheeses, plain or with chives

1 large egg, beaten

75 g/3 oz/1½ cups cornflakes, crushed

175 g/6 oz mixed salad leaves

45 ml/3 tbsp cranberry sauce

45 ml/3 tbsp olive oil

15 ml/1 tbsp red wine vinegar

Freshly ground black pepper

Oil, for shallow-frying

---

1 Cut each of the goats' cheeses into four slices and dip the slices in egg, then crushed cornflakes. Repeat so that they are well coated. Chill for at least 1 hour.

2 Arrange the salad leaves in small piles on individual plates.

3 Whisk the cranberry sauce, oil and vinegar together with plenty of freshly ground black pepper,

4 Shallow-fry the cheeses quickly for 2–3 minutes until golden brown and crisp on the outside, turning over once. Drain on kitchen paper (paper towels).

5 Place on top of the salad and drizzle the dressing over. Serve immediately.

Parma-style Aubergines

If you can't tolerate the Parmesan cheese, garnish with a few thin strips of anchovy fillet.

SERVES 4

---

2 large aubergines (eggplants), diced

25 g/1 oz/2 tbsp unsalted (sweet) butter

30 ml/2 tbsp olive oil

2 red onions, thinly sliced

100 g/4 oz pancetta, finely diced

400 g/14 oz/1 large can of chopped tomatoes

5 ml/1 tsp dried basil

2.5 ml/½ tsp balsamic vinegar

Salt and freshly ground black pepper

50 g/2 oz Parmesan cheese, cut into thin shavings with a potato peeler

1 Boil the aubergine cubes in salted water for 5 minutes. Drain and dry on kitchen paper (paper towels).

2 Heat the butter and oil in a flameproof casserole (Dutch oven). Add the onions and fry (sauté), stirring, for 2 minutes. Add the pancetta and fry for a further 2 minutes.

3 Add the tomatoes, bring to the boil, reduce the heat and simmer for 5 minutes, stirring occasionally, until pulpy.

4 Add the aubergines, basil and balsamic vinegar. Cover and simmer very gently for 30 minutes until the aubergines are soft and richly bathed in sauce.

5 Serve hot, sprinkled with the Parmesan cheese.

Westphalian Ham and Celeriac Salad

SERVES 4

1 celeriac (celery root)

5 ml/1 tsp lemon juice

30 ml/2 tbsp Cooked Mayonnaise (see page 181 or buy gluten-free mayonnaise)

10 ml/2 tsp caraway seeds

A few drops of Tabasco sauce

2.5 ml/½ tsp white wine vinegar

Salt and freshly ground black pepper

8 slices of Westphalian raw ham

1 Peel the celeriac and cut into fairly thin slices, then cut each slice into thin matchsticks.

2 Boil in plenty of salted water to which the lemon juice has been added for 3 minutes. Drain, rinse with cold water and drain again.

3 Mix the Cooked Mayonnaise with half the caraway seeds, the Tabasco, vinegar and seasoning. Add the celeriac and toss well. Chill for 30 minutes to allow the flavours to develop.

4 Arrange the slices of ham attractively on four plates with the celeriac salad. Sprinkle the salad with the remaining caraway seeds before serving.

Creamy Scallops with Oyster Mushrooms

If you can get scallops in their shells, scrub the deep halves of the shells and serve this dish in them instead of individual flameproof dishes. Substitute finely chopped, salted peanuts for the Parmesan and soya yoghurt for the crème fraîche if you are lactose intolerant.

SERVES 4

450 g/1 lb potatoes, peeled and cut into small pieces

15 ml/½ oz/1 tbsp butter or margarine

275 ml/ 9 fl oz/scant 1¼ cups milk

4 scallops, cleaned

1 bay leaf

1 slice of onion

100 g/4 oz oyster mushrooms, sliced

30 ml/2 tbsp cornflour (cornstarch)

60 ml/4 tbsp crème fraîche

Salt and freshly ground black pepper

30 ml/2 tbsp grated Parmesan cheese

30 ml/2 tbsp crushed cornflakes

25 g/1 oz/2 tbsp butter or margarine, melted

4 small sprigs of parsley, to garnish

1 Boil the potatoes in lightly salted water until really tender. Drain thoroughly, mash, then beat in the butter or margarine and 30 ml/2 tbsp of the milk until light and fluffy.

2 Either spoon the potato around the edge of four individual flameproof serving dishes or put into a piping bag fitted with a large star tube (tip) and pipe a border of potato in each dish.

3 Rinse the scallops and cut into quarters.

4 Bring all but 30 ml/2 tbsp of the remaining milk, the bay leaf and onion to the boil and simmer for 3 minutes. Strain into a clean pan. Add the mushrooms, cover and cook gently for 4 minutes. Add the scallops and cook for a further 3 minutes.

5 Lift out the scallops and mushrooms with a draining spoon and place in the centres of the prepared dishes.

6 Blend the cornflour with the remaining milk and add to the cooking milk. Bring to the boil and cook, stirring, for 1 minute until thickened.

7 Stir in the crème fraîche and salt and pepper to taste. Spoon over the scallops and mushrooms.

8 Mix the Parmesan and cornflakes together and sprinkle over the sauce. Brush the tops gently with melted butter or margarine. Place the dishes under a preheated moderate grill (broiler) and cook for a few minutes until lightly browning. Garnish with parsley and serve hot.

Spiced Chicken Livers with Rocket and Mango

SERVES 4

1 ripe mango

1 onion, very finely chopped

30 ml/2 tbsp olive oil

45 ml/3 tbsp apple juice

5 ml/1 tsp garam masala

225 g/8 oz chicken livers, trimmed and cut into bite-sized pieces

Salt and freshly ground black pepper

15 ml/1 tbsp chopped fresh coriander (cilantro)

100 g/4 oz rocket

Lemon juice, to taste

1 Peel the mango and slice the flesh in neat pieces off the stone (pit).

2 Fry (sauté) the onion gently in half the olive oil for 3 minutes, stirring, until softened but not browned.

3 Add 30 ml/2 tbsp of the apple juice and the garam masala and simmer, stirring, until the liquid has almost evaporated.

4 Add the chicken livers and a little salt and pepper and cook, stirring, for 3–4 minutes until the chicken livers are just cooked but still soft. Stir in the coriander.

5 Arrange the rocket and mango slices on four plates.

6 Whisk the remaining olive oil and apple juice together with a little salt, pepper and lemon juice, to taste. Drizzle over the salads.

7 Spoon the livers on top and serve straight away.

Rustic Liver Pâté

SERVES 6

350 g/12 oz pigs' liver, cut into chunks

400 g/14 oz fat streaky bacon, rinded

1 onion, quartered

1 cooking (tart) apple, cored and quartered

150 ml/¼ pt/⅔ cup water

1.5 ml/¼ tsp dried sage

Salt and freshly ground black pepper

15 ml/1 tbsp brandy (optional)

50 g/2 oz/¼ cup butter, melted

2 bay leaves and a few juniper berries, to garnish

Toasted wheat-free/gluten-free bread (buy ready-made or see pages 155–7) or Sesame Crackers (see page 159), to serve

1 Mince (grind) the liver, bacon, onion and apple finely or chop finely in a blender or food processor, dropping in a piece at a time with the machine running.

2 Place in a saucepan with the water, sage and a little salt and pepper. Bring to the boil, cover, reduce the heat and cook gently for 25 minutes, stirring occasionally.

3 Turn the mixture into a 900 ml/1½ pt/3¾ cup serving dish and press down well.

4 Leave until cold, then place a double thickness of greaseproof (waxed) paper over the top and weigh down with heavy weights or cans of food. Chill until firm.

5 Pour the melted butter over and garnish with bay leaves and juniper berries. Chill until set. Serve with wheat-free/gluten-free toast or Sesame Crackers.

Potato Pan Pizza

If you are lactose intolerant, you may not be able to tolerate the cheese. If so, omit it altogether and cover the top with a mixture of 25 g/1 oz/2 tbsp smooth peanut butter and 25 g/ 1 oz/2 tbsp soya spread before grilling (broiling).

SERVES 2–4

---

225 g/8 oz potatoes, peeled and cut into chunks

25 g/1 oz/2 tbsp butter or margarine

75 g/3 oz/¾ cup rice flour, plus a little for dusting

2.5 ml/½ tsp gluten-free baking powder

A good pinch of salt

A little milk

15 ml/1 tbsp sunflower or olive oil

30 ml/2 tbsp tomato purée (paste)

3 tomatoes, sliced

2.5 ml/½ tsp dried oregano

75 g/3 oz/¾ cup Cheddar or Mozzarella cheese, grated

A few black olives

---

1 Boil the potatoes in lightly salted water until tender. Drain and return to the pan.

2 Mash well with the butter or margarine and work in the rice flour, baking powder, a good pinch of salt and enough milk to form a firm dough.

3 Roll out on a surface dusted with rice flour to a round the size of the base of a fairly large frying pan (skillet).

4 Heat the oil in the frying pan and add the potato. Cook for about 2 minutes until the base is golden brown. Tip out of the pan on to a large, flameproof plate, then slide back in, with the browned side up. Cook for a

further 2–3 minutes until browned underneath.

5 Slide out on to the plate again. Spread with the tomato purée, then top with the tomatoes, oregano and cheese and sprinkle with a few olives. Place under a preheated grill (broiler) until the cheese has melted and is browning slightly. Serve hot.

Onion Bhajis

SERVES 4

75 g/3 oz/¾ cup gram flour

75 ml/5 tbsp water

2.5 ml/½ tsp chilli powder

1.5 ml/¼ tsp ground turmeric

5 ml/1 tsp ground coriander (cilantro)

5 ml/1 tsp salt

Sunflower oil, for deep-frying

15 ml/1 tbsp chopped fresh coriander

2 onions, halved and thinly sliced

1 Mix the flour with the water to make a fairly stiff batter, adding a dash more water if necessary.

2 Mix in the spices and salt and beat until smooth. Leave to stand for 30 minutes.

3 Heat the oil to 190°C/375°F or until a cornflake dropped in rises to the surface and sizzles immediately.

4 Meanwhile, mix the coriander and onion into the batter. Shape into small, rough balls, drop into the hot oil and cook for about 5 minutes until golden. Drain on kitchen paper (paper towels).

Mushroom and Basil Tartlets

Ring the changes by using a little chopped ham or bacon instead of mushrooms. Turn the tartlets into a main meal by adding a Potato and Yoghurt Salad (see pages 130–31) and some crisp salad vegetables. If you are lactose intolerant, omit the cheese if necessary and add a little extra seasoning and 30 ml/2 tbsp extra (soya) milk.

MAKES 12

⅓ quantity of Savoury Pastry (see page 175)

Rice flour, for dusting

1 egg

4 button mushrooms, thinly sliced

5 ml/1 tsp dried minced (ground) onion

30 ml/2 tbsp water

60 ml/4 tbsp milk

Salt and freshly ground black pepper

10 ml/2 tsp chopped fresh basil

50 g/2 oz/½ cup Cheddar cheese, grated

1   Roll out the pastry (paste) on a surface dusted with rice flour and cut into 12 rounds using a 7.5 cm/3 in biscuit (cookie) cutter.

2   Press into the 12 sections of a tartlet tin (patty pan). Break the egg into a small bowl. Dip a pastry brush into the white and brush all over the pastry cases (pie shells).

3   Bake in a preheated oven at 200°C/400°F/gas mark 6 for 10 minutes or until set and turning golden.

4   Meanwhile, put the mushrooms, onion and water in a small bowl and cook in the microwave on High for 1 minute. Alternatively, place in a saucepan, cover and simmer gently for 3 minutes until soft.

5 Spoon the mushroom mixture (without any liquid) into the pastry cases.

6 Beat the milk into the remaining egg and season. Stir in the basil. Pour over the mushrooms.

7 Top with the cheese. Bake in the oven for about 15 minutes until set and golden. Cool slightly, then remove from the tin and serve warm or cold.

Tortilla

SERVES 4

2 large potatoes, very thinly sliced

1 large onion, very thinly sliced

45 ml/3 tbsp olive oil

6 eggs

Salt and freshly ground black pepper

1 Fry (sauté) the potatoes and onion very gently in the olive oil for about 8–10 minutes, stirring and turning frequently, until softened but not browned.

2 Spread out evenly in the pan. Beat the eggs with a little salt and pepper and pour into the pan. Cook gently, lifting the edge to allow the uncooked egg to run underneath until the base is set and golden.

3 Place the pan under a moderate preheated grill (broiler) and cook until set. Serve hot or cold, cut into wedges.

Home-made Burgers

Those with wheat intolerance can use bought dill pickles as can coeliacs who can tolerate malt or spirit vinegar.

SERVES 4

---

225 g/8 oz lean minced (ground) beef, lamb, pork, chicken or turkey

5 ml/1 tsp dried onion granules

5 ml/1 tsp dried mixed herbs

Salt and freshly ground black pepper

1 egg, beaten

A little sunflower oil

8 fairly thick slices of wheat-free/gluten-free bread, preferably Milk Loaf (see page 156)

Gluten-free tomato ketchup (catsup)

4 Dill Pickled Cucumber Slices (see page 184)

1 small onion, finely chopped

A little shredded lettuce

---

1 Mix the minced meat or poultry with the onion granules, herbs and a little salt and pepper.

2 Stir in the beaten egg to bind, then shape the mixture into four flat cakes.

3 Place on foil on a grill (broiler) rack and brush with a little oil. Grill (broil) for about 3–4 minutes on each side until golden brown and cooked through.

4 Cut the largest rounds possible from the bread slices, using a biscuit (cookie) cutter. (Save the crusts for crumbs for a separate recipe.)

5 Spread four slices with a little ketchup and top each with a burger. Top the burgers with a Dill Pickled Cucumber Slice, a little chopped onion and shredded lettuce. Top with the second slices of bread and serve.

Asparagus Omelette

SERVES 4

4 eggs

60 ml/4 tbsp cold water

Salt and freshly ground black pepper

5 ml/1 tsp dried oregano

25 g/1 oz/2 tbsp butter or margarine

295 g/10½ oz/1 medium can of asparagus spears, drained

A little Chilli Salsa (see page 186), optional

1 Beat one of the eggs in a bowl with 15 ml/1 tbsp of the water, a little salt and pepper and a quarter of the oregano.

2 Heat 10 ml/¼ oz/2 tsp of the butter or margarine in a small non-stick frying pan (skillet). Add the egg mixture and fry (sauté) lifting the edge of the mixture to allow the uncooked egg to run underneath.

3 When the base is set and golden, slide out of the pan, then turn back in and cook for a further minute to set the other side. Slide out and leave to cool while cooking the remaining 3 eggs in the same way.

4 Divide the asparagus spears between the four omelettes. Top with a little Chilli Salsa, if liked, roll up and eat in your fingers.

Sausage Rolls

These are delicious served with Sweet Chutney (see page 185)
and some tomatoes and cucumber.

MAKES ABOUT 14–16

⅓ quantity of Savoury Pastry (see page 175)

Rice flour, for dusting

½ quantity of sausagemeat (see page 30)

Beaten egg, to glaze

1 Cut the pastry (paste) in half. On a surface dusted liberally with rice flour, roll out each piece to an oblong about 10 cm/4 in wide.

2 Cut the sausagemeat in half and shape each into a long sausage the same length as the pieces of pastry. Lay each sausage on a piece of pastry, towards one side.

3 Brush the edges with beaten egg and gently fold the pastry over the sausagemeat and press the edges together.

4 Knock up the long edges. Mark lines across the top diagonally to decorate, then cut each length into seven or eight pieces.

5 Transfer to a non-stick baking (cookie) sheet and brush the tops with beaten egg to glaze.

6 Bake in a preheated oven at 200°C/400°F/gas mark 6 for about 20 minutes until golden and cooked through. Transfer to a wire rack. Serve warm or cold.

Cheese Soufflé

If you can't tolerate the cheese – or if you just fancy a change – make a Tuna Soufflé. Omit the cheese and beat a drained 185 g/6½ oz/small can of tuna and 15 ml/1 tbsp tomato purée (paste) into the cornflour (cornstarch) mixture.

SERVES 2–4

30 ml/2 tbsp cornflour

150 ml/¼ pt/⅔ cup milk

25 g/1 oz/2 tbsp butter or margarine, plus a little for greasing

3 eggs, separated

100 g/4 oz/1 cup strong Cheddar cheese, grated

A good pinch of cayenne

Salt and freshly ground black pepper

1 Blend the cornflour with the milk in a saucepan and add the butter or margarine. Bring to the boil, stirring, until thick.

2 Beat in the egg yolks and cheese and add the cayenne and some salt and pepper.

3 Whisk the egg whites until stiff and fold in with a metal spoon.

4 Turn into a greased 15 cm/6 in soufflé dish and bake in a preheated oven at 190°C/375°F/gas mark 5 for about 25–30 minutes until well risen, golden and just set. Serve straight away.

MEAT AND POULTRY
MAIN MEALS

Main meals aren't quite such a problem
– you can grill (broil), fry (sauté) or
roast any meat or poultry and as long
as you thicken any accompanying
sauces with cornflour (cornstarch)
instead of ordinary flour, you'll be fine.
To add variety, however, I thought it
would be a good idea to give you some
ideas for main courses that would
otherwise be banished from your diet –
like a scrumptious version of Chicken
Maryland, without the usual
breadcrumb coating (see page 69).
These versions of popular favourites are
just as good as their originals – and in
some cases, I think they're even better.

Chicken Maryland

4 chicken portions

30 ml/2 tbsp cornflour (cornstarch)

Salt and freshly ground black pepper

1 egg, beaten

50 g/2 oz plain potato crisps (chips), fairly finely crushed

50 g/2 oz/¼ cup butter or margarine

60 ml/4 tbsp sunflower oil

4 small bananas

A little lemon juice

Oven-sautéed Potatoes with Garlic (see page 124), Corn Fritters (see page 125) and a green salad, to serve

1 Wipe the chicken and toss in the cornflour, seasoned with a little salt and pepper.

2 Dip the chicken in the beaten egg and then the crisps until well coated.

3 Heat 40 g/1½ oz/3 tbsp of the butter or margarine and 45 ml/3 tbsp of the oil in a roasting tin (pan). Add the chicken and turn over in the fat. Roast in a preheated oven at 200°C/400°F/gas mark 6 for about 45 minutes until golden and cooked through.

4 Meanwhile, halve the bananas and toss in a little lemon juice. Melt the remaining butter or margarine and the remaining oil in a small roasting tin and add the bananas. Turn over in the fat, then roast beside the chicken for about 20 minutes until cooked through.

5 Serve the chicken with the bananas, Oven-sautéed Potatoes with Garlic, Corn Fritters and a green salad.

Millet Couscous with Garlic Chicken

SERVES 4

100 g/4 oz/1 cup millet grains

4 chicken portions

50 g/2 oz/¼ cup butter or margarine

1 garlic clove, crushed

Salt and freshly ground black pepper

1 red (bell) pepper, chopped

1 red onion, chopped

400 g/14 oz/1 large can of chopped tomatoes

30 ml/2 tbsp tomato purée (paste)

30 ml/2 tbsp red wine

5 ml/1 tsp caster (superfine) sugar

50 g/2 oz stoned (pitted) black olives

A few torn coriander (cilantro) leaves, to garnish

1 Boil the millet in plenty of lightly salted water for about 20 minutes until tender.

2 Drain in a colander, rinse with boiling water and drain again. Place the colander over a saucepan of hot water over a gentle heat, to keep the grains warm until ready to serve.

3 Meanwhile, place the chicken portions, skin-sides down, on foil on a grill (broiler) rack.

4 Melt the butter or margarine in a medium saucepan and add the garlic and a little salt and pepper. Brush over the chicken and grill (broil) for 10 minutes.

5 Turn the chicken over, brush liberally with the garlic butter again and grill for a further 15–20 minutes until cooked through and golden brown.

6 While the chicken is grilling, cook the red pepper and onion for 3 minutes in the remaining garlic butter in the saucepan. Add the tomatoes, tomato purée, wine, sugar and olives and simmer, stirring occasionally, for about 6 minutes until pulpy.

7 When everything is cooked, spoon the cooked millet on to four warm plates. Place a pool of the sauce to one side and top with a piece of chicken. Scatter a few torn coriander leaves over and serve hot.

Chicken Satay

1 small onion, finely chopped

1 garlic clove, crushed

15 ml/1 tbsp sunflower oil

30 ml/2 tbsp smooth peanut butter

10 ml/2 tsp lemon juice

15 ml/1 tbsp clear honey

15 ml/1 tbsp gluten-free soy sauce

1.5 ml/¼ tsp chilli powder

120 ml/4 fl oz/½ cup milk

450 g/1 lb chicken fillets, cubed

Lemon wedges, to garnish

Wild Rice Salad (see page 131), to serve

1 Fry (sauté) the onion and garlic in a saucepan in the oil for 2 minutes to soften.

2 Stir in all the remaining ingredients except the milk and chicken and bring to the boil, stirring.

3 Stir in 90 ml/6 tbsp of the milk, reduce the heat and simmer gently, stirring, for 2 minutes.

4 Thread the chicken on to soaked wooden skewers. Brush with a little of the sauce.

5 Place on foil on a grill (broiler) rack and grill (broil) for about 8 minutes, turning frequently and brushing with more sauce.

6 Thin the remaining sauce with the remaining milk and reheat, then spoon into small pots. Put the chicken on warm plates with the small pots of sauce. Garnish with lemon wedges and serve with a Wild Rice Salad.

French Chicken with Beans

SERVES 4

30 ml/2 tbsp olive oil

25 g/1 oz/2 tbsp butter or margarine

450 g/1 lb baby potatoes, scrubbed

4 chicken portions

100 g/4 oz chestnut mushrooms, sliced

Salt and freshly ground black pepper

200 ml/7 fl oz/scant 1 cup gluten-free chicken stock

100 g/4 oz French (green) beans, topped and tailed and cut into short lengths

2 garlic cloves, chopped

30 ml/2 tbsp chopped fresh parsley

1 Heat half the oil and half the butter or margarine in a large frying pan (skillet). Add the potatoes and cook, tossing, until browned all over. Remove from the pan.

2 Heat the remaining oil and butter or margarine in the pan and brown the chicken thoroughly on all sides.

3 Return the potatoes to the pan and add the mushrooms and some salt and pepper. Pour in 60 ml/ 4 tbsp of the stock. Cover and cook over a gentle heat for 45 minutes until the chicken and potatoes are tender.

4 Meanwhile, cook the beans in a little boiling, lightly salted water for 4 minutes until just tender. Drain.

5 Add the beans to the chicken mixture and scatter the garlic and parsley over. Re-cover and continue to cook for 5 minutes. Transfer everything to a warm platter.

6 Add the remaining stock to the pan, stir and boil for 1 minute, scraping up any residue in the pan. Spoon over the chicken and serve.

Minted Lemon-glazed Chicken

SERVES 4

---

4 chicken portions

30 ml/2 tbsp cornflour (cornstarch)

Salt and freshly ground black pepper

50 g/2 oz/¼ cup butter or margarine

30 ml/2 tbsp sunflower oil

Finely grated rind and juice of 1 small lemon

1 small onion, grated

2.5 ml/½ tsp dried mint

10 ml/2 tsp caster (superfine) sugar

Sprigs of parsley, to garnish

Mustard Seed Potatoes (see page 124) and broccoli, to serve

1 Wipe the chicken. Mix the cornflour with a little salt and pepper and dust all over the chicken.

2 Melt the butter or margarine in a roasting tin (pan). Add the chicken, skin-sides down, and roast in a preheated oven at 180°C/350°F/gas mark 4 for 20 minutes. Turn the portions over and roast for a further 20 minutes.

3 Whisk the oil, lemon, onion, mint and sugar together with a little salt and pepper. Spoon over the chicken and cook for a further 15–20 minutes, basting once or twice until tender, golden and stickily glazed.

4 Transfer to warm plates and garnish with parsley.

5 Spoon off all the excess fat from the juices in the tin. Add 30 ml/2 tbsp boiling water and stir well. Season to taste. Spoon over the chicken and serve with Mustard Seed Potatoes and broccoli.

Crunchy Turkey Escalopes

This recipe works equally well with pork steaks.

SERVES 4
---

4 turkey breast steaks

75 g/3 oz/¾ cup millet flakes

15 ml/1 tbsp dried minced (ground) onion

5 ml/1 tsp dried sage

15 ml/1 tbsp chopped fresh parsley

Salt and freshly ground black pepper

1 egg, beaten

Sunflower oil, for frying (sautéing)

Lemon wedges and sprigs of parsley, to garnish

Creamed potatoes and Cauliflower and Broccoli Cheese (see page 123), to serve

1 Put the turkey steaks one at a time in a plastic bag and beat with a rolling pin or meat mallet until flattened.

2 Mix the millet with the dried onion, sage and parsley. Season well with salt and pepper.

3 Dip each escalope first in beaten egg and then in the millet mixture to coat well.

4 Heat the oil in a large frying pan (skillet) and fry the turkey for about 3 minutes on each side until golden brown and cooked through. Drain on kitchen paper (paper towels).

5 Transfer to warm plates, garnish with lemon wedges and sprigs of parsley and serve hot with creamed potatoes and Broccoli and Cauliflower Cheese.

Turkey and Asparagus Stir-fry with Soba Noodles

Buy packs of asparagus pieces if you can – they are a lot cheaper.

SERVES 4

---

350 g/12 oz thin asparagus spears, cut into two pieces

350 g/12 oz turkey steaks, cut into thin strips

1 large leek, cut into thin shreds

45 ml/3 tbsp sunflower oil

200 g/7 oz/1 small can of pimientos, drained and sliced

100 g/4 oz button mushrooms, sliced

90 ml/6 tbsp apple juice

45 ml/3 tbsp gluten-free soy sauce

2.5 cm/1 in piece of fresh root ginger, grated

Salt and freshly ground black pepper

250 g/9 oz 100% buckwheat soba noodles

---

1 Boil the asparagus in lightly salted water for 3 minutes. Drain.

2 Stir-fry the turkey and leek in the oil for 2 minutes. Add the pimientos and mushrooms and stir-fry for a further 2 minutes.

3 Add the asparagus and all the remaining ingredients except the noodles and stir-fry for 2 minutes. Cover, reduce the heat and cook for a further 5 minutes.

4 Meanwhile, boil the noodles in lightly salted water for 5 minutes. Drain and rinse with boiling water. Drain again. Spoon on to warm plates. Top with the turkey mixture and serve straight away.

Lamb Medallions with Rosemary and Port

SERVES 4

350 g/12 oz lamb neck fillet, cut into 12 slices

Salt and freshly ground black pepper

25 g/1 oz/2 tbsp butter or margarine

15 ml/1 tbsp olive oil

1 small onion, very finely chopped

15 ml/1 tbsp finely chopped fresh rosemary

30 ml/2 tbsp redcurrant jelly (clear conserve)

60 ml/4 tbsp port

120 ml/4 fl oz/½ cup gluten-free vegetable stock

15 ml/1 tbsp tomato purée (paste)

Sprigs of rosemary, to garnish

Creamed potatoes and Spring Greens with Celery (see page 123), to serve

1 Put the lamb slices in a plastic bag, one at a time, and beat with a rolling pin or meat mallet, to flatten. Season with salt and pepper.

2 Fry (sauté) the slices in the butter or margarine and oil for about 2 minutes on each side until brown and just cooked. Remove from the pan and keep warm.

3 Put the onion in the pan and fry, stirring, for 2–3 minutes to soften. Add the remaining ingredients and stir until blended. Bring to the boil and simmer for 2 minutes. Taste and re-season, if necessary.

4 Transfer the lamb to warm plates. Pour any juices into the sauce, then spoon over the lamb and garnish with sprigs of rosemary. Serve with creamed potatoes and Spring Greens with Celery.

Curried Turkey and Avocado Salad

Check the curry powder you buy has no wheat flour added to prevent clumping. Use soya yoghurt instead of crème fraîche if you are lactose intolerant.

SERVES 4

30 ml/2 tbsp sunflower oil

1 onion, grated

10 ml/2 tsp curry powder

5 ml/1 tsp ground turmeric

15 ml/1 tbsp lemon juice

30 ml/2 tbsp gluten-free mango chutney

45 ml/3 tbsp crème fraîche

30 ml/2 tbsp milk

225 g/8 oz/2 cups cooked turkey, diced

1 ripe avocado, diced

1 red eating (dessert) apple, diced

4 poppadoms

A little extra sunflower oil

Sprigs of coriander (cilantro), to garnish

1 Heat the oil in a frying pan (skillet) and fry (sauté) the grated onion, stirring, for 1 minute. Add the curry powder and turmeric and fry for a further 30 seconds.

2 Tip into a bowl and stir in the lemon juice, mango chutney, crème fraîche and milk.

3 Fold in the turkey, avocado and apple.

4 Shallow-fry the poppadoms in a little sunflower oil until they curl up round the edges but are not brown. Drain on kitchen paper (paper towels). Leave to cool.

5   When ready to serve, place the poppadoms on four plates. Pile salad on each and garnish with sprigs of coriander.

Corned Beef Stuffed Pancakes

If you are lactose intolerant, use Béchamel Sauce (see page 179) and omit the grated cheese if necessary.

SERVES 4

---

1 quantity of Brittany Pancakes (see page 174)

350 g/12 oz/1 medium can of corned beef, cut into chunks

45 ml/3 tbsp gluten-free tomato ketchup (catsup)

A few drops of Tabasco sauce

1 quantity of Cheese Sauce (see page 178)

50 g/2 oz/½ cup Cheddar cheese, grated

4 tomatoes, sliced

---

1   Make the pancakes and keep warm.

2   Put the corned beef in a saucepan with the tomato ketchup and Tabasco sauce. Heat through gently, stirring until piping hot.

3   Divide between the pancakes and roll up. Place in a shallow, flameproof dish.

4   Spoon the cheese sauce over and sprinkle with the cheese. Arrange the tomato slices around the edge.

5   Grill (broil) until golden and bubbling. Serve hot.

Lamb Biryani

1 onion, sliced

15 ml/1 tbsp sunflower oil

225 g/8 oz/2 cups cooked lamb, diced

1 garlic clove, crushed

2.5 ml/½ tsp ground ginger

2.5 ml/½ tsp ground cumin

2.5 ml/½ tsp ground coriander (cilantro)

7.5 ml/1½ tsp ground turmeric

150 ml/¼ pt/⅔ cup plain yoghurt

Salt and freshly ground black pepper

225 g/8 oz/1 cup basmati rice

2.5 cm/1 in piece of cinnamon stick

4 cardamom pods, split

45 ml/3 tbsp toasted flaked (slivered) almonds

30 ml/2 tbsp currants

30 ml/2 tbsp chopped fresh coriander

Gluten-free mango chutney, to serve

1 Fry (sauté) the onion in the oil for 3 minutes until lightly golden.

2 Add the lamb, garlic, ground ginger, cumin and coriander, 2.5 ml/½ tsp of the ground turmeric and the yoghurt. Sprinkle with salt and pepper. Simmer for 20 minutes, stirring occasionally until the mixture is almost dry (it will curdle and separate at first).

3 Meanwhile, boil the rice in plenty of lightly salted water, to which the remaining turmeric, the cinnamon stick and cardamom pods have been added, for about 10 minutes or until just tender. Drain. Remove the cinnamon and cardamom.

4 Spoon the rice on to four warm plates. Top with the lamb mixture. Mix the almonds, currants and chopped coriander together and sprinkle over. Serve with mango chutney.

Buckwheat Lasagne al Forno

You can cut the pasta into thin shreds and boil in lightly salted water for 4–5 minutes, then drain and serve with the Bolognese sauce as Tagliatelle Bolognese, if you prefer. Alternatively, use the sauce with any bought wheat-free/gluten-free pasta. If you are lactose intolerant, use Béchamel Sauce (see page 179) instead of Cheese Sauce and omit the Parmesan if necessary.

SERVES 4

75 g/3 oz/¾ cup buckwheat flour

A pinch of salt

1 large egg, beaten

Cornflour (cornstarch), for dusting

1 onion, finely chopped

1 garlic clove, crushed

1 carrot, finely chopped

350 g/12 oz minced (ground) beef or lamb

400 g/14 oz/1 large can of chopped tomatoes

15 ml/1 tbsp tomato purée (paste)

30 ml/2 tbsp red wine (optional)

5 ml/1 tsp caster (superfine) sugar

Freshly ground black pepper

5 ml/1 tsp dried oregano

1½ quantities of Cheese Sauce (see page 178)

15 ml/1 tbsp grated Parmesan cheese

A green salad, to serve

1 Put the buckwheat flour and salt in a bowl.

2 Add the egg and work with a fork until a ball of dough is forming, then knead together with the hands. Turn out on to a board and knead until fairly smooth. Wrap and leave to rest for 15 minutes.

3 Roll out thinly on a board dusted with cornflour. Cut into six sheets about 7.5 × 15 cm/3 × 6 in, re-kneading and rolling the trimmings as necessary. Leave to dry on the board while you prepare the Bolognese sauce.

4 Put the onion, garlic, carrot and meat in a saucepan and dry-fry, stirring all the time, until all the grains of meat are separate and no longer pink.

5 Add the tomatoes, tomato purée, wine, if using, sugar, some salt and pepper and the oregano. Bring to the boil, stirring, reduce the heat and simmer for 15 minutes.

6 Put a spoonful of the meat sauce in the base of a shallow 1.2 litre/2 pt/5 cup ovenproof dish. Top with two sheets of lasagne. Layer half the remaining meat, two more sheets of pasta, the remaining meat and the remaining pasta. Cover with the cheese sauce and sprinkle with the Parmesan cheese.

7 Bake in a preheated oven at 190°C/375°F/gas mark 5 for about 35–40 minutes until golden and cooked through. Serve hot with a green salad.

Chilli con Carne with Crispy Tacos

If you are lactose intolerant, omit the cheese if necessary and add a finely chopped avocado, tossed with a few drops of Tabasco sauce, and use soya yoghurt instead of soured cream.

SERVES 4

225 g/8 oz minced (ground) beef or lamb

1 large onion, finely chopped

2.5 ml/½ tsp chilli powder

5 ml/1 tsp ground cumin

5 ml/1 tsp dried oregano

300 ml/½ pt/1¼ cups passata (sieved tomatoes)

15 ml/1 tbsp tomato purée (paste)

425 g/15 oz/1 large can of red kidney beans, undrained

Salt and freshly ground black pepper

12 crispy corn taco shells

¼ iceberg lettuce, shredded

100 g/4 oz/1 cup Cheddar cheese, grated

150 ml/¼ pt/⅔ cup soured (dairy sour) cream, to serve

1 Put the meat, onion, chilli powder, cumin and oregano in a saucepan. Cook, stirring, until the grains of meat are separate and no longer pink.

2 Add the passata, tomato purée, the can of kidney beans and some salt and pepper. Stir well. Bring to the boil, reduce the heat and simmer for 20 minutes until a rich sauce is formed. Taste and re-season if necessary.

3 Meanwhile, warm the taco shells as directed on the packet. Line with shredded lettuce.

4 Spoon the chilli into the shells, top with a little cheese and soured cream and serve straight away.

Middle Eastern Grilled Supper

If you are lactose intolerant, you may be able to eat Halloumi cheese, made with sheep's milk. If not, substitute slices of aubergine (eggplant) instead, cooking until golden and tender.

SERVES 4

---

150 ml/¼ pt/⅔ cup plain yoghurt

5 cm/2 in piece of cucumber, peeled

1 small garlic clove, crushed

Salt and freshly ground black pepper

5 ml/1 tsp dried mint

1 quantity of sausages (see page 30)

200 g/7 oz/1 block of Halloumi cheese, cut into 8 slices

A little olive oil

Lemon wedges and sprigs of parsley, to garnish

Quinoa Tabbouleh (see page 129), to serve

1 Put the yoghurt in a bowl.

2 Grate the cucumber and squeeze to remove excess moisture. Stir into the yoghurt with the garlic, a little salt and pepper and the mint. Chill until ready to serve.

3 Grill (broil) the sausages on foil on a grill (broiler) rack for about 6 minutes, turning once or twice until golden and cooked through. After 3 minutes, add the Halloumi cheese slices to the grill rack, brush with oil and grill for about 1½ minutes each side until just turning golden.

4 Transfer the sausages and Halloumi to warm plates. Put a spoonful of the yoghurt dip to one side and garnish the plates with lemon wedges and sprigs of parsley. Serve with Quinoa Tabbouleh.

Polish Stuffed Cabbage

SERVES 4

8 large cabbage leaves

175 g/6 oz minced (ground) beef

50 g/2 oz/¼ cup long-grain rice

Salt and freshly ground black pepper

30 ml/2 tbsp tomato purée (paste)

30 ml/2 tbsp chopped fresh parsley

1 garlic clove, crushed

2.5 ml/½ tsp dried mixed herbs

Approx 1 litre/1¾ pts/4¼ cups gluten-free beef or vegetable stock

4 smoked streaky bacon rashers (slices), rinded

Potato and Yoghurt Salad (see pages 130–31), to serve

1 Cut out the thick central base of the stalk from each cabbage leaf. Blanch the leaves in boiling water for 3 minutes. Drain, rinse with cold water, drain again and dry on kitchen paper (paper towels).

2 Mix together the beef, rice, some salt and pepper, the tomato purée, half the parsley, the garlic and the mixed herbs.

3 Spoon the mixture into the centre of each cabbage leaf, fold in the sides and roll up. Pack in a single layer in a flameproof casserole (Dutch oven).

4 Pour over enough stock to cover. Bring to the boil, cover, reduce the heat and simmer very gently for 1½ hours, adding a little more stock if necessary during cooking.

5 Meanwhile, grill (broil) the bacon until crisp and snip into pieces with scissors.

6 Transfer the stuffed cabbage on to warm plates. Boil the stock in the casserole until syrupy and spoon over the cabbage. Sprinkle with the remaining parsley and the bacon. Serve with a Potato and Yoghurt Salad.

Nasi Goreng

SERVES 4

350 g/12 oz/1½ cups long-grain rice

1 bunch of spring onions (scallions), roughly chopped

1 large garlic clove, crushed

1 green chilli, seeded and chopped

4 canned anchovy fillets

75 ml/5 tbsp sunflower oil

225 g/8 oz pork fillet, cut into thin strips

15 ml/1 tbsp gluten-free soy sauce

4 eggs

1 Cook the rice in plenty of boiling, lightly salted water for 10 minutes until just tender. Drain, rinse with cold water and drain again.

2 Purée the spring onions, garlic, chilli and anchovies with 60 ml/4 tbsp of the oil in a blender or food processor.

3 Spoon the purée into a large frying pan (skillet) and fry (sauté) for 30 seconds. Add the pork and stir-fry for about 5 minutes until cooked through. Add the rice and continue cooking for a few minutes, tossing until glistening and piping hot. Stir in the soy sauce.

4 Meanwhile, fry the eggs in a separate pan in the remaining oil. Pile the rice on to warm plates and top with the eggs.

Steak, Kidney and Mushroom Pie

Ideally, cook the meat the day before the pie is required.

SERVES 4
450 g/1 lb lean stewing beef, diced
100 g/4 oz ox kidney, diced
1 large onion, chopped
2 carrots, sliced
1 bay leaf
Freshly ground black pepper
1 gluten-free beef stock cube
15 ml/1 tbsp gluten-free soy sauce
100 g/4 oz button mushrooms, sliced
45 ml/3 tbsp cornflour (cornstarch)
½ quantity of Savoury Pastry (see page 175)
Beaten egg or plain yoghurt, to glaze
New potatoes and Spring Greens with Celery (see page 123), to serve

1 Put the meat, kidney, onion, carrots, bay leaf and a little pepper in a saucepan. Add just enough water to cover and stir in the stock cube and soy sauce. Bring to the boil, skim the surface, reduce the heat, part-cover and simmer gently for 2 hours until the meat is tender. Add the mushrooms for the last 5 minutes.

2 Blend the cornflour with 45 ml/3 tbsp water and stir into the liquid in the pan. Cook, stirring, for 1 minute, to thicken. Remove the bay leaf and leave to cool.

3 Turn the meat and some of the gravy into a 1.5 litre/ 2½ pt/6 cup pie dish with a pie funnel or upturned ceramic eggcup in the centre.

4 Roll out the pastry (paste) until it is a little larger than the pie dish and cut a strip off the edge all round. Brush the edge of the pie dish with water and lay the pastry strip on this. Brush with water again.

5 Lay the pastry over the top, making a small cut in the centre where the pie funnel is to allow the steam to escape.

6 Knock up the edge and flute with the back of a knife, or press all round with the prongs of a fork.

7 Brush with beaten egg or yoghurt, to glaze, and bake in a preheated oven at 200°C/400°F/gas mark 6 for about 40 minutes until golden brown. Reheat any remaining gravy.

8 Serve hot with the remaining gravy, new potatoes and Spring Greens with Celery.

Pork and Bean Cassoulet

All dried beans should be soaked for several hours, preferably overnight, and then boiled rapidly for 10 minutes, to remove any toxins, before simmering until tender.

SERVES 4

225 g/8 oz/1½ cups dried haricot (navy) beans

Boiling water

450 ml/¾ pt/2 cups cold water

1 gluten-free vegetable stock cube

15 ml/1 tbsp sunflower oil

350 g/12 oz belly pork, rinded and diced

2 onions, chopped

2 carrots, chopped

1 turnip, diced

225 g/8 oz/1 small can of chopped tomatoes

15 ml/1 tbsp black treacle (molasses)

1 bay leaf

Salt and freshly ground black pepper

30 ml/2 tsp chopped fresh parsley, to serve

---

1 Cover the beans with boiling water and leave to soak for several hours. Drain and place in a large, flameproof casserole (Dutch oven). Add the measured water, bring to the boil and boil rapidly for 10 minutes. Stir in the stock cube.

2 Meanwhile, heat the oil in a frying pan (skillet) and add the pork and onions. Fry (sauté) for 3 minutes until lightly golden.

3 Add to the beans with all the remaining ingredients and stir well.

4 Cover and place in a preheated oven at 150°C/300°F/ gas mark 2 for 4 hours or until the beans are really tender and bathed in a rich sauce. Discard the bay leaf, taste and re-season if necessary.

5 Sprinkle with chopped parsley and serve in warm bowls.

Pork Schnitzels

If you cannot tolerate Mozzarella cheese, substitute slices of firm tofu.

SERVES 4

8 thin pork escalopes, about 350 g/12 oz in all

2 thin slices of ham, halved

100 g/4 oz Mozzarella cheese, thinly sliced

45 ml/3 tbsp potato flour

Salt and freshly ground black pepper

1 large egg, beaten

50 g/2 oz/1 cup cornflakes, crushed

A little sunflower oil

Garlic and Herb Bread Slices (see page 176) and Grilled Sweet Peppers with Olives and Sunflower Seeds (see page 132), to serve

1 Put the escalopes in a plastic bag, one at a time, and beat with a rolling pin or meat mallet to flatten.

2 Sandwich the escalopes together in pairs with half a slice of ham and a little sliced cheese.

3 Press well together, then dust with potato flour seasoned with salt and pepper.

4 Dip in the beaten egg and then the cornflakes, to coat completely.

5 Heat enough oil to cover the base of a large frying pan (skillet). Fry (sauté) the schnitzels for about 4 minutes on each side until golden brown and cooked through.

6 Drain on kitchen paper (paper towels), then serve hot with Garlic and Herb Bread Slices and Grilled Sweet Peppers with Olives and Sunflower Seeds.

Plum Barbecued Spare Ribs

SERVES 4

---

15 g/½ oz/1 tbsp butter or margarine

10 ml/2 tsp sesame oil

1 small onion, finely chopped

1 garlic clove, crushed

2.5 cm/1 in piece of fresh root ginger, grated

5 ml/1 tsp ground cumin

60 ml/4 tbsp plum jam (conserve)

15 ml/1 tbsp red wine vinegar

30 ml/2 tbsp gluten-free soy sauce

30 ml/2 tbsp medium sherry

450 g/1 lb pork spare ribs

Far Eastern Salad (see page 133), to serve

---

1 Heat the butter or margarine with the oil in a saucepan and fry (sauté) the onion for 2 minutes.

2 Add the garlic, ginger and cumin and fry for a further 1 minute.

3 Stir in the jam, vinegar, soy sauce and sherry.

4 Place the ribs in a shallow dish and pour the sauce over. Leave to marinate for at least 2 hours, turning occasionally.

5 Place on foil on a grill (broiler) rack, lay the ribs on this and grill (broil) for 15–20 minutes, turning occasionally and basting with the sauce until tender, cooked through and stickily glazed. Serve hot with a Far Eastern Salad.

Honey Roast Ham in Cider

It is always best to bring a gammon joint to the boil in water before use, to be sure that it is not too salty.

SERVES 6

---

700 g /1½ lb unsmoked gammon joint

300 ml/½ pt/1¼ cups medium cider

150 g/¼ pt/⅔ cup water

Freshly ground black pepper

6 cloves

30 ml/2 tbsp clear honey

45 ml/3 tbsp cornflour (cornstarch)

5 ml/1 tsp dried mixed herbs

Mustard Seed Potatoes (see page 124) and Cauliflower and Broccoli Cheese (see page 123), to serve

---

1 Put the joint in a saucepan and cover with water. Bring to the boil and discard the water.

2 Place the joint in a roasting tin (pan) and pour the cider and measured water around. Sprinkle the joint with pepper.

3 Cover with a lid or foil and roast in a preheated oven at 190°C/375°F/gas mark 5 for 1 hour.

4 Remove the lid or foil and cut or pull off any rind on the joint. If there is any fat, score it in a criss-cross pattern. Stud the surface with the cloves. Mix the honey with 15 ml/1 tbsp of the cornflour, the herbs and a good grinding of pepper and smear over the surface of the joint.

5 Return, uncovered, to the oven and cook for a further 20–25 minutes until golden brown.

6 Transfer to a carving dish. Blend the remaining cornflour with 30 ml/2 tbsp water and add to the juices. Bring to the boil and cook, stirring, for 1 minute, until thickened slightly. Taste and re-season if necessary.

7 Carve the joint and serve with the sauce, Mustard Seed Potatoes and Cauliflower and Broccoli Cheese.

FISH AND VEGETABLE MAIN COURSES

You can, of course, eat any amount of grilled (broiled), baked or fried (sautéed) fish – as long as it isn't coated in flour, breadcrumbs or ordinary batter before cooking. All the pulses – dried peas, beans and lentils – are ideal too. However, many vegetarian recipes include large quantities of wholemeal flour or breadcrumbs for added nutritional value which, of course, you must avoid. Here is a selection of my favourite fish and vegetarian recipes, all carefully adapted to exclude wheat and gluten. You can even tuck into traditional fish and chips – see page 121 for a recipe with the crispiest batter ever!

Seafood Pie with Mushrooms

SERVES 4

450 g/1 lb potatoes, scrubbed and thinly sliced

350 g/12 oz white fish fillet, skinned

450 ml/¾ pt/2 cups milk

100 g/4 oz button mushrooms, sliced

Salt and freshly ground black pepper

5 ml/1 tsp dried thyme

30 ml/2 tbsp chopped fresh parsley

225 g/8 oz frozen seafood cocktail, thawed

30 ml/2 tbsp cornflour (cornstarch)

15 g/½ oz/1 tbsp butter or margarine, melted

Mangetout (snow peas), to serve

1 Cook the sliced potatoes in boiling, lightly salted water for 4 minutes until just tender but still holding their shape. Drain.

2 Meanwhile, cut the white fish into cubes, discarding any bones. Place in a saucepan with all but 30 ml/ 2 tbsp of the milk and the mushrooms. Bring to the boil and simmer for 4 minutes until the fish is almost tender. Season and stir in the thyme and parsley. Add the seafood and cook for a further 2 minutes.

3 Blend the cornflour with the remaining milk and stir into the fish. Bring to the boil and cook, stirring very gently, for 1 minute until thickened.

5 Turn into a 1.2 litre/2 pt/5 cup flameproof dish. Top with the sliced potatoes and brush with the butter or margarine. Grill (broil) for about 5–6 minutes until golden brown. Serve hot with mangetout.

Warm Grilled Salmon and Citrus Salad

SERVES 4

4 salmon steaks

45 ml/3 tbsp pure orange juice

90 ml/6 tbsp olive oil

2 grapefruit

2 oranges

175 g/6 oz mixed salad leaves

2 carrots, coarsely grated

1 bunch of spring onions (scallions), trimmed and cut into short lengths

8 radishes, sliced

15 ml/1 tbsp lemon juice

5 ml/1 tsp chopped fresh oregano

5 ml/1 tsp clear honey

Salt and freshly ground black pepper

New potatoes, to serve

1 Put the steaks, skin-sides down, on foil on a grill (broiler) rack. Mix 15 ml/1 tbsp each of the pure orange juice and the oil and brush over the fish. Grill (broil) for 7–8 minutes until cooked through. Do not turn over.

2 Meanwhile, holding the fruit over a bowl to catch the juice, cut all the peel and pith off the grapefruit and oranges and cut the fruit into segments. Squeeze the membranes to extract the last of the juice.

3 Toss the salad leaves, carrots, spring onions and radishes together and pile on to plates.

4 Whisk the remaining pure orange juice and oil in the bowl with the grapefruit and orange juice and whisk in the lemon juice, oregano, honey and salt and pepper to taste. Spoon over the salads and arrange the orange and grapefruit segments around.

5 Top each with a salmon steak and serve with new potatoes.

Mackerel in Millet

If you are wheat intolerant, you can use oatmeal instead of millet for a change.

SERVES 4

---

4 mackerel, cleaned

75 g/3 oz/¾ cup millet flakes

30 ml/2 tbsp chopped fresh parsley

5 ml/1 tsp paprika

Salt and freshly ground black pepper

1 egg, beaten

60 ml/4 tbsp sunflower oil

Lemon wedges and sprigs of parsley, to garnish

New potatoes and Blushing Butter Beans (see page 126), to serve

---

1 Rinse the fish and dry on kitchen paper (paper towels). Trim the fins and cut off the tails. Split all the way along the stomach. Open out and place skin-sides up on a board. Run the thumb up and down the centre of the back to loosen the backbone of each fish. Turn over and remove the backbone and any loose bones.

2 Mix the millet with the parsley, paprika and a little salt and pepper. Dip the fish in the beaten egg and then the millet mixture to coat completely.

3 Brush a baking (cookie) sheet with some of the oil. Add the fish, skin-sides down. Drizzle with the remaining oil. Bake near the top of a preheated oven at 190°C/ 375°F/gas mark 5 for about 25 minutes until golden and cooked through. Transfer to warm plates.

4 Garnish with lemon wedges and parsley and serve with new potatoes and Blushing Butter Beans.

Soused Herrings with Apple

You can try this with mackerel too.

SERVES 4

---

4 herrings, cleaned and heads removed

2 small onions

1 eating (dessert) apple, finely chopped

5 ml/1 tsp dried dill (dill weed)

15 ml/1 tbsp pickling spices

1 bay leaf

120 ml/4 fl oz/½ cup cider vinegar

120 ml/4 fl oz/½ cup water

15 ml/1 tbsp light brown sugar

1.5 ml/¼ tsp salt

Potato and Yoghurt Salad (see pages 130–31), to serve

---

1 Lay the fish flat on a board, skin-sides up. Run your thumb firmly up and down the backbone of each several times, to loosen it. Turn over and lift off the backbone and all the loose bones.

2 Finely chop one of the onions. Scatter over the fish with the apple and sprinkle with the dill. Roll up and place in an ovenproof dish.

3 Slice the remaining onion and scatter over with the pickling spices. Add the bay leaf.

4 Mix the remaining ingredients together and pour over. Cover with foil and bake in a preheated oven at 160°C/325°F/gas mark 3 for 1 hour until the fish is cooked through. Leave to cool in the liquid, then chill before serving with Potato and Yoghurt Salad.

Paella

Saffron powder, which is traditionally used in paella for colouring and flavour, is very expensive. Ground turmeric makes an excellent cheap alternative.

SERVES 6

---

6 chicken thighs

60 ml/4 tbsp olive oil

1 onion, finely chopped

100 g/4 oz pancetta or rindless streaky bacon, diced

1 red (bell) pepper, diced

1 green pepper, diced

350 g/12 oz/1½ cups paella or risotto rice

450 g/1 lb mussels in their shells, scrubbed and beards removed

Approx 1 litre/1¾ pts/4¼ cups gluten-free chicken or vegetable stock

5 ml/1 tsp saffron powder or ground turmeric

2 ripe tomatoes, skinned, seeded and chopped

100 g/4 oz frozen peas

Salt and freshly ground black pepper

1 bay leaf

5 ml/1 tsp dried marjoram

100 g/4 oz cooked peeled prawns (shrimp)

Lemon wedges

6 whole cooked prawns

30 ml/2 tbsp chopped fresh parsley

1 Brown the chicken thighs for 10 minutes in the oil in a paella pan or very large frying pan (skillet). Remove from the pan.

2 Add the onion and pancetta or bacon and fry (sauté) for 3 minutes until softened and lightly browned.

3 Add the peppers and rice and cook, stirring, for 1 minute. Return the chicken to the pan. Add the mussels and enough stock to cover the ingredients. Stir in the saffron or turmeric, tomatoes, peas and a little salt and pepper and add the bay leaf and marjoram.

4 Bring to the boil, reduce the heat, cover and simmer gently for 20 minutes or until the rice is cooked and has absorbed most of the liquid. Add a little more stock during cooking if necessary.

5 Remove the mussels. Snap off the top shells and discard any mussels that have not opened. Keep the mussels warm in the bottom shells. Stir the peeled prawns into the rice mixture and heat through. Return the mussels to the pan and garnish with the lemon wedges, whole prawns and chopped parsley. Serve piping hot.

Plaice with Tomato and Corn Rice

If the skin on your plaice fillets is white, it is soft and edible.
Remove any skin that is black before use.

SERVES 4

175 g/6 oz/¾ cup long-grain rice

400 g/14 oz/1 large can of chopped tomatoes

300 ml/½ pt/1¼ cups water

Salt and freshly ground black pepper

200 g/7 oz/1 small can of sweetcorn (corn)

15 ml/1 tbsp chopped fresh parsley

8 plaice fillets

2 eggs, beaten

100 g/4 oz/1 cup cornmeal

A little sunflower oil

Sprigs of parsley and lemon wedges, to serve

1 Put the rice in a saucepan with the tomatoes, water and some salt and pepper. Bring to the boil, reduce the heat, cover and simmer gently for 20 minutes until the rice is tender and has absorbed all the liquid. Stir in the sweetcorn and parsley and heat through.

2 Meanwhile, dip the fish fillets in beaten egg and then in the cornmeal, seasoned with a little salt and pepper, to coat completely. Repeat to give a good coating.

3 Heat a little oil in a large frying pan (skillet) and fry (sauté) the plaice fillets for 2–3 minutes on each side until golden brown and cooked through. Drain on kitchen paper (paper towels) and keep warm while cooking the remaining fish.

4 Pile the rice on warm plates, top with the fish and garnish with sprigs of parsley and lemon wedges.

Halibut Parcels

Try this with salmon or cod steaks too.

SERVES 4

15 ml/1 tbsp olive oil

2 courgettes (zucchini), thinly sliced

50 g/2 oz button mushrooms, thinly sliced

25 g/1 oz/2 tbsp butter or margarine

4 halibut steaks, about 175 g/6 oz each

Finely grated rind and juice of 1 small lemon

Freshly ground black pepper

50 g/2 oz/1 small can of anchovy fillets, drained

30 ml/2 tbsp chopped fresh parsley

1 hard-boiled (hard-cooked) egg, finely chopped

New potatoes and mangetout (snowpeas), to serve

1 Brush four large squares of foil with the oil. Arrange the courgettes over the centre of each in a single layer. Lay the mushrooms on top.

2 Dot with half the butter or margarine, then place a fish steak on top of each. Sprinkle with the lemon rind and juice and a good grinding of pepper.

3 Lay the anchovies in a criss-cross pattern over each fish fillet and dot with the remaining butter or margarine. Loosely wrap in the foil, sealing the edges together well.

4 Transfer to a baking (cookie) sheet and bake for about 30 minutes in a preheated oven at 190°C/375°F/gas mark 5 until tender.

5 Carefully open up each parcel, slide the fish on to warm plates and sprinkle with the chopped parsley and egg. Serve hot with new potatoes and mangetout.

Grilled Tuna with Lentils

*Try this with marlin or swordfish steaks for a change, and use
a lime or an orange instead of the lemon.*

SERVES 4

---

175 g/6 oz/1 cup green lentils

60 ml/4 tbsp sunflower oil

1 red onion, finely chopped

1 bouquet garni sachet

Finely grated rind and juice of 1 lemon

Approx 600 ml/1 pt/2½ cups gluten-free vegetable stock

Salt and freshly ground black pepper

50 g/2 oz/¼ cup butter, softened

30 ml/2 tbsp chopped fresh parsley

4 tuna steaks

Tomato and Onion Salad (see page 127), to serve

1 Soak the lentils in cold water for 2 hours, then drain.

2 Heat half the oil in a saucepan. Add the onion and
   cook gently for 3 minutes until softened but not
   browned.

3 Add the lentils, bouquet garni, lemon rind and juice
   and enough vegetable stock to cover. Bring to the boil,
   reduce the heat and simmer for 25–30 minutes until
   tender and most of the liquid has been absorbed.
   Season to taste.

4 Meanwhile, mash the butter with the parsley and a
   little pepper and divide into four pats.

5 Place the tuna steaks on foil on the grill (broiler) rack. Brush with oil and season lightly. Grill (broil) for about 3 minutes on each side until cooked through and tender. Do not overcook. Place a pat of flavoured butter on each steak and return to the grill until it starts to melt. Remove immediately.

6 Spoon the lentils on to warm plates. Set the tuna steaks on top and serve with a Tomato and Onion Salad.

Tuna and Sweetcorn Pancakes

If you are lactose intolerant, use Béchamel Sauce (see page 179) and omit the cheese if necessary.

SERVES 4
1 quantity of Brittany Pancakes (see page 174)
1 quantity of Cheese Sauce (see page 178)
185 g/6½ oz/1 small can of tuna, drained
200 g/7 oz/1 small can of sweetcorn (corn), drained
30 ml/2 tbsp chopped fresh parsley
50 g/2 oz/½ cup Cheddar cheese, grated
Sliced cucumber and tomatoes in Vinaigrette Dressing (see page 183), to serve

1 Make up the pancakes and keep warm.

2 Make the cheese sauce and stir in the tuna, corn and parsley and heat through.

3 Divide between the pancakes and roll up. Place in a shallow, flameproof dish.

4 Sprinkle with the cheese and place under a preheated grill (broiler) until golden and bubbling. Serve hot with sliced cucumber and tomatoes, tossed in Vinaigrette Dressing.

Nutty Cheese Cod

*If you are lactose intolerant, substitute 25 g/1 oz/2 tbsp
peanut butter for the cheese if necessary and use peanuts
instead of walnuts.*

SERVES 4

40 g/1½ oz/3 tbsp butter or margarine

4 pieces of cod fillet, about 175 g/6 oz each, skinned

Freshly ground black pepper

50 g/2 oz/½ cup Cheddar cheese, grated

15 ml/1 tbsp plain yoghurt

30 ml/2 tbsp chopped walnuts

2 spring onions (scallions), finely chopped

3–4 tomatoes, sliced

Plain boiled potatoes and peas, to serve

1 Grease a large flameproof dish with a little of the butter
   or margarine and lay the fish in a single layer in the
   dish, skinned sides up.

2 Dot with 15 ml/½ oz/1 tbsp of the butter or margarine
   and sprinkle with pepper. Grill (broil) for 2 minutes.
   Turn over.

3 Mash the remaining butter or margarine with the
   cheese, yoghurt, walnuts and spring onions and add a
   little pepper. Spread all over the fish. Reduce the heat
   and grill for a further 7–8 minutes or until bubbling,
   golden and cooked through.

4 Arrange the tomatoes around the edge and grill for a
   few extra minutes. Serve hot with plain boiled potatoes
   and peas.

Cottage Garden Pie

You can use cooked, leftover vegetables in this dish. Boil the rice alone for the full 10 minutes, and then add the vegetables, chopped into small pieces, with the beans. Omit the cheese if you can't tolerate it.

SERVES 4

50 g/2 oz/¼ cup long-grain rice

350 g/12 oz frozen mixed vegetables

450 g/1 lb potatoes, peeled and cut into small pieces

15 g/½ oz/1 tbsp butter or margarine

30 ml/2 tbsp milk

400 g/14 oz/1 large can of gluten-free baked beans

10 ml/2 tsp yeast extract

30 ml/2 tbsp boiling water

Salt and freshly ground black pepper

75 g/3 oz/¾ cup Cheddar cheese, grated

1 Cook the rice in plenty of boiling, salted water in a flameproof casserole (Dutch oven) for 3 minutes. Add the mixed vegetables and cook for a further 7 minutes until just tender. Drain and return to the casserole. Chop or snip with scissors.

2 Meanwhile, boil the potatoes in a separate pan of salted water until tender. Drain and mash with the butter or margarine and milk.

3 Stir the beans into the rice mixture. Dissolve the yeast extract with the boiling water and stir into the vegetable mixture. Season to taste.

4 Spread the mashed potato over the top and sprinkle with the cheese. Bake in a preheated oven at 220°C/425°F/gas mark 7 for 35 minutes until golden.

Potato Gnocchi

Omit the Parmesan cheese if you can't tolerate it.

SERVES 4

---

450 g/1 lb potatoes, peeled and cut into chunks

Salt and freshly ground black pepper

1.5 ml/¼ tsp grated nutmeg

50 g/2 oz/½ cup soya flour

50 g/2 oz/½ cup potato flour, plus extra for dusting

1 egg, beaten

50 g/2 oz/¼ cup butter or margarine, melted

Grated Parmesan cheese and chopped fresh basil, to garnish

Warmed passata (sieved tomatoes), Courgette Coleslaw (see page 130) and a crisp green salad, to serve

---

1   Boil the potatoes in lightly salted water until tender. Drain and return to the pan over a gentle heat for a minute or two to dry out. Mash thoroughly with a little salt, lots of pepper and the nutmeg.

2   Beat in the flours and then the egg to form a soft dough. Knead gently on a surface dusted with potato flour until no longer sticky. Roll into about 30 small balls.

3   Bring a large pan of water to the boil and cook the gnocchi in two batches for about 5 minutes until they rise to the surface. Remove and transfer to a warm serving dish, greased with a little of the butter or margarine. Keep warm while cooking the remainder.

4   Drizzle the melted butter or margarine over and sprinkle liberally with Parmesan cheese and basil. Serve with warmed passata, Courgette Coleslaw and a crisp, green salad.

Grilled Polenta with Cheese and Basil

If you can't tolerate the cheese, substitute ground hazelnuts (filberts).

SERVES 4

---

900 ml/1½ pts/3¾ cups water

5 ml/1 tsp salt

225 g/8 oz/2 cups polenta

75 g/3 oz/⅓ cup butter or margarine

75 g/3 oz/¾ cup Parmesan cheese, grated

15 ml/1 tbsp chopped fresh basil

60 ml/4 tbsp olive oil

Sprigs of basil, to garnish

Tomato and Onion Salad (see page 127), to serve

---

1 Put the water and salt in a non-stick saucepan and bring to the boil.

2 Gradually stir in the polenta and cook until it begins to thicken. Reduce the heat and simmer very gently for 20 minutes, stirring occasionally, until really thick.

3 Stir in the butter or margarine, 50 g/2 oz/½ cup of the cheese and the chopped basil.

4 Brush a shallow baking tin (pan) with a little of the oil and add the polenta, smoothing out to about 2.5 cm/ 1 in thick. Leave until cold, then chill.

5 When ready to cook, cut the polenta into 5 cm/2 in squares. Place on foil on a grill (broiler) rack and brush with the remaining oil. Grill (broil) for 5 minutes, then turn over and brush with more oil. Continue to grill until golden brown.

6 Transfer to warm plates, sprinkle with the remaining cheese and garnish with basil sprigs. Serve with a Tomato and Onion Salad.

Cannelloni with Spinach and Tofu

If you can't tolerate the cheese, omit it and cover the dish with foil before baking.

SERVES 4

175 g/6 oz/1½ cups buckwheat flour

A good pinch of salt

2 large eggs, beaten

Cornflour (cornstarch), for dusting

350 g/12 oz frozen chopped spinach, thawed

297 g/11 oz/1 block of firm tofu, drained

1.5 ml/¼ tsp grated nutmeg

5 ml/1 tsp dried mixed herbs

Freshly ground black pepper

400 g/14 oz/1 large can of chopped tomatoes

100 g/4 oz/1 cup Cheddar cheese, grated

Chicory, Orange and Cashew Nut Salad (see page 128), to serve

1 Put the flour and salt in a bowl. Add the eggs and work with a fork until the mixture is forming a dough, then knead together with the hands. Knead until fairly smooth, then cover and leave to stand for 15 minutes.

2 Cut into two pieces. Roll out each piece as thinly as possible on a surface dusted with cornflour. Cut each into six strips about 7.5 × 15 cm/3 × 6 in, re-kneading and rolling the trimmings as necessary.

3 Mash the spinach and tofu together with the nutmeg, herbs and some salt and pepper. Spoon on to the strips and roll up to form stuffed tubes. Place, seam-sides down, in a single layer in a shallow ovenproof dish.

4   Cover with the tomatoes and then the cheese. Bake in a preheated oven at 190°C/375°F/gas mark 5 for about 35 minutes until golden brown and cooked through. Serve hot with a Chicory, Orange and Cashew Nut Salad.

Dutch Rice Supper

If you are lactose intolerant, omit the cheese if necessary, add a layer of chopped ham in the middle and pour 2 beaten eggs over before adding the cornflakes.

SERVES 4

---

175 g/6 oz/¾ cup long-grain rice

25 g/1 oz/2 tbsp unsalted (sweet) butter

2 large onions, chopped

225 g/8 oz/2 cups Edam cheese, grated

4 tomatoes, sliced

Freshly ground black pepper

30 ml/2 tbsp cornflakes, crushed

A green salad, to serve

---

1   Cook the rice according to the packet directions. Drain, rinse with cold water and drain again.

2   Meanwhile, melt half the butter and fry (sauté) the onions for 3 minutes until lightly golden.

3   Grease a 1.5 litre/2½ pt/6 cup ovenproof dish with the remaining butter. Put a layer of half the cooked rice in the dish. Add half the onions and half the cheese and cover with the remaining rice. Top with the remaining onions, then the tomatoes and season. Cover with the remaining cheese and the cornflakes.

4   Bake in a preheated oven at 190°C/375°F/gas mark 5 for about 30 minutes until piping hot and turning golden. Serve hot with a green salad.

Falafels

MAKES 8–10

1 large onion, quartered

425 g/15 oz/1 large can of chick peas (garbanzos), drained

1 garlic clove, crushed

5 ml/1 tsp ground coriander (cilantro)

5 ml/1 tsp ground cumin

5 ml/1 tsp caraway seeds

10 ml/2 tsp chopped fresh parsley

2.5 ml/½ tsp gluten-free baking powder

1 egg, separated

50 g/2 oz/1 cup cornflakes, finely crushed

A little sunflower oil

Cresmolto Salad (see pages 126–7), to serve

1 Drop the onion into a food processor with the machine running and roughly chop.

2 Add the chick peas and garlic and run the machine until fairly smooth, stopping and scraping down the sides if necessary.

3 Add the coriander, cumin, caraway seeds, parsley, baking powder, egg yolk and just enough milk to bind the mixture together without making it 'wet'.

4 Shape into small balls. Roll in the lightly beaten egg white and then the cornflakes. Repeat the coating to cover thoroughly and chill for at least 30 minutes.

5 Shallow-fry in hot oil, turning once until crisp and golden. Drain on kitchen paper (paper towels). Serve warm with a Cresmolto Salad.

Mushroom and Artichoke Pilau

SERVES 4

1 onion, finely chopped

1 garlic clove, crushed

30 ml/2 tbsp sunflower oil

2.5 cm/1 in piece of fresh root ginger, grated

175 g/6 oz button mushrooms, sliced

1.5 ml/¼ tsp garam masala

225 g/8 oz/1 cup basmati rice

400 ml/14 fl oz/1¾ cups gluten-free vegetable stock

425 g/15 oz/1 large can of artichoke hearts, quartered

Salt and freshly ground black pepper

30 ml/2 tbsp chopped fresh coriander (cilantro), to garnish

Carrot, Courgette and Yellow Pepper Salad (see pages 128–9), to serve

1 Fry (sauté) the onion and garlic in the oil for 3 minutes until lightly golden.

2 Stir in the ginger, mushrooms, garam masala and rice and stir until every grain of rice is glistening.

3 Add the stock, artichoke hearts and some salt and pepper. Stir gently and bring to the boil.

4 Cover with foil, then a saucepan lid, to seal tightly. Reduce the heat to as low as possible and leave to cook for 20 minutes. Turn off the heat and leave to stand, undisturbed, for 5 minutes.

5 Remove the lid and foil, fluff up the pilau with a fork and serve, sprinkled with the coriander, with a Carrot, Courgette and Yellow Pepper Salad.

Hot Potato and Quorn Sauté

175 g/6 oz Quorn pieces

30 ml/2 tbsp gluten-free soy sauce

15 ml/1 tbsp medium sherry

1 garlic clove, crushed

700 g/1½ lb new potatoes, scraped or scrubbed and cut into even-sized pieces

50 g/2 oz/¼ cup butter or margarine

30 ml/2 tbsp sunflower oil

1 bunch of spring onions (scallions), cut into short lengths

1 green (bell) pepper, cut into thin strips

1 red pepper, cut into thin strips

350 g/12 oz/1 large can of sweetcorn (corn), drained

2.5 ml/½ tsp dried oregano

10 ml/2 tsp paprika

30 ml/2 tbsp chopped fresh parsley

Tomato and Onion Salad (see page 127), to serve

1 Put the Quorn in a shallow dish. Mix the soy sauce, sherry and garlic together and pour over. Toss well and leave to marinate for 1 hour.

2 Meanwhile, boil the potatoes in lightly salted water for about 8–10 minutes until just tender. Drain.

3 Melt the butter or margarine and the oil in a large frying pan (skillet). Add the spring onions and peppers and fry (sauté), stirring, for 2 minutes. Add the potatoes and cook, tossing lightly, for about 5 minutes.

4 Add the Quorn, sweetcorn, oregano and paprika and continue to toss gently over the heat for 5 minutes.

5 Pile on to warm plates, sprinkle with parsley and serve with a Tomato and Onion Salad.

Quinoa and Aubergine Sandwiches

SERVES 4

2 small aubergines (eggplants)

Salt

175 g/6 oz/1 cup quinoa, rinsed

1.75 litres/3 pts/7½ cups water

100 g/4 oz/1 cup cornmeal

15 ml/1 tbsp peanut butter

Freshly ground black pepper

75 g/3 oz/¾ cup salted peanuts, finely chopped

1 garlic clove, crushed

30 ml/2 tbsp chopped fresh parsley

1.5 ml/¼ tsp cayenne

Olive oil, for brushing

200 ml/7 fl oz/scant 1 cup passata (sieved tomatoes)

2.5 ml/½ tsp dried basil

5 ml/1 tsp caster (superfine) sugar

Cresmolto Salad (see pages 126–7), to serve

1 Cut the stalks off the aubergines, then cut each one lengthways into four thick slices. Sprinkle with salt and place in a colander. Leave to stand while making the filling.

2 Cook the quinoa for about 20 minutes in 1.2 litres/ 2 pts/5 cups of the water with a pinch of salt added, until tender and it has absorbed the liquid. Season with pepper.

3 In a separate pan, bring the remaining water to the boil. Add the cornmeal, peanut butter and a little salt and pepper. Cook, stirring frequently, over a gentle heat for about 3 minutes until very thick and the mixture leaves the sides of the pan clean. Stir in the peanuts and leave to cool.

4 Combine the two mixtures with the garlic, parsley and cayenne. Shape into four oval patties, just smaller than the aubergine slices.

5 Rinse the aubergine slices and pat dry on kitchen paper (paper towels). Place on a grill (broiler) rack with the patties and brush everything with oil. Grill (broil) for about 10 minutes, turning once until cooked and golden brown.

6 Warm the passata in a saucepan with the basil, sugar and some salt and pepper.

7 Put an aubergine slice on each of four warm plates. Top with a patty and then another aubergine slice. Spoon the passata over and serve with a Cresmolto Salad.

Veggie Cheese Burgers

If you can't tolerate the cheese, substitute chopped, mixed nuts.

SERVES 4
1 potato, cut into small pieces
1 parsnip, cut into small pieces
1 carrot, cut into small pieces
25 g/1 oz/2 tbsp butter or margarine
Freshly ground black pepper
75 g/3 oz/¾ cup Cheddar cheese, grated
200 g/7 oz/1 small can of sweetcorn (corn)
50 g/2 oz frozen peas, thawed
A few drops of Tabasco sauce
Salt, to taste
1 egg, beaten
50 g/2 oz/1 cup cornflakes, crushed
Sunflower oil
Chilli Salsa (see page 186) and a mixed salad, to serve

1 Boil the potato, parsnip and carrot together in lightly salted water until really tender. Drain and mash with the butter or margarine and some pepper.

2 Beat in the cheese and stir in the sweetcorn, peas and a few drops of Tabasco. Season with salt if necessary.

3 Shape into eight small cakes, dip in beaten egg and then cornflakes to coat completely. Chill, if time allows.

4 Brush with oil and place on foil on a grill (broiler) rack. Grill (broil) for about 4 minutes on each side until golden. Serve with Chilli Salsa and a mixed salad.

Traditional English Fish 'n' Chips

4 good-sized potatoes, scrubbed or peeled

Sunflower oil

40 g/1½ oz/⅓ cup cornflour (cornstarch)

40 g/1½ oz/⅓ cup rice flour

A good pinch of salt

15 ml/1 tbsp gluten-free baking powder

105–120 ml/7–8 tbsp water

4 fillets of cod or haddock, about 175 g/6 oz each, skinned

Lemon wedges, to garnish

Peas and Tartare Sauce (see page 182), to serve

1 Cut the potatoes into thick slices, then slice these into fingers. Place in a bowl of cold water and soak for at least 5 minutes. Drain and dry.

2 Heat about 2.5 cm/1 in sunflower oil in a large frying pan (skillet). Slide the chips (fries) down a fish slice held against the side of the pan.

3 Fry (sauté) the chips for about 8 minutes, turning once or twice until crisp and golden. Drain on kitchen paper (paper towels).

4 Mix the flours with the salt and baking powder and stir in enough water to form a thick, creamy batter.

5 Heat another pan with oil to a depth of about 5 mm/ ¼ in. Dip the fish in the batter and place in the pan. Cook for about 3 minutes on each side until crisp, golden and cooked through. Drain on kitchen paper.

6 Garnish the fish and chips with lemon wedges on warm plates and serve with peas and Tartare Sauce.

VEGETABLE AND SALAD SIDE DISHES

The recipes in this section offer perfect ways to brighten up plain-cooked meat, fish or poultry. They can also be used to accompany the main-course recipes in this book.

Cauliflower and Broccoli Cheese

If you can't tolerate cheese, use Béchamel Sauce (page 179).

SERVES 4

½ small cauliflower, cut into small florets

175 g/6 oz broccoli, cut into small florets

1 quantity of Cheese Sauce (see page 178)

30 ml/2 tbsp crushed cornflakes

1 Boil the cauliflower and broccoli in lightly salted water for about 4 minutes until just tender but still with some bite. Drain well and turn into a flameproof dish.

2 Pour the Cheese Sauce over and top with the crushed cornflakes.

3 Grill (broil) until golden and bubbling.

Spring Greens with Celery

SERVES 4
---

3 celery sticks, sliced

450 ml/¾ pt/2 cups gluten-free vegetable stock

350 g/12 oz spring (collard) greens, shredded

1 Put the celery sticks in a fairly large saucepan with the stock. Bring to the boil, cover, reduce the heat and simmer for 5 minutes.

2 Add the spring greens, press down well, and boil rapidly, uncovered, for about 4–5 minutes, stirring occasionally, until the vegetables are just tender and the liquid has evaporated. Serve hot.

Mustard Seed Potatoes

You can cook these for a slightly shorter time in a hotter oven if that is more convenient.

SERVES 4

700 g/1½ lb potatoes, scrubbed and halved or quartered

30 ml/2 tbsp olive oil

Salt and freshly ground black pepper

30 ml/2 tbsp black mustard seeds

1 Put the potato pieces in a roasting tin (pan). Pour the oil over and toss to coat completely.

2 Season with salt and pepper and sprinkle with the mustard seeds.

3 Roast towards the top of a preheated oven at 180°C/350°F/gas mark 4 for 1½ hours or until golden brown and tender, turning once during cooking.

Oven-sautéed Potatoes with Garlic

SERVES 4

700 g/1½ lb potatoes, scrubbed and diced

45 ml/3 tbsp olive oil

40 g/1½ oz/3 tbsp butter or margarine

1–2 garlic cloves, finely chopped

Salt

1 Put the diced potatoes in a bowl of cold water until ready to cook.

2 Drain and dry on kitchen paper (paper towels). Heat the oil and butter or margarine in a baking tin (pan). Add the potatoes and toss to coat completely. Add the garlic and a little salt and toss again.

3 Bake near the top of a preheated oven at 200°C/400°F/ gas mark 6 for about 45 minutes, turning two or three times, until golden brown and cooked through. Drain on kitchen paper and serve hot.

Corn Fritters

These are good served with Aioli (see page 182) as a starter or with bacon for breakfast and are wonderful as a side dish with any grilled (broiled), fried (sautéed) or roasted meat or poultry. You can also make fritters using mushrooms, blanched broccoli or cauliflower florets or leftover, cooked mixed vegetables instead of sweetcorn (corn).

SERVES 4

40 g/1½ oz/⅓ cup rice flour

40 g/1½ oz/⅓ cup cornflour (cornstarch)

A good pinch of salt

15 ml/1 tbsp gluten-free baking powder

105–120 ml/7–8 tbsp water

200 g/7 oz/1 small can of sweetcorn, drained

60 ml/4 tbsp sunflower oil

1 Mix the flours with the salt and baking powder and stir in the water to form a thick, creamy batter.

2 Stir in the sweetcorn.

3 Heat the oil in a frying pan (skillet) and add spoonfuls of the batter. Fry until golden brown underneath. Turn over and cook until golden and crisp. Drain on kitchen paper (paper towels). Serve hot.

Blushing Butter Beans

SERVES 4
---

1 onion, chopped

30 ml/2 tbsp olive oil

1 garlic clove, crushed

225 g/8 oz/1 small can of chopped tomatoes

A pinch of caster (superfine) sugar

Salt and freshly ground black pepper

425 g/15 oz/1 large can of butter (lima) beans, drained

15 ml/1 tbsp snipped fresh chives, to garnish

1 Cook the onion gently in the oil for 3 minutes until softened but not browned.
2 Add all the remaining ingredients, stir gently and simmer for 5 minutes.
3 Sprinkle with the chives and serve hot.

Cresmolto Salad

SERVES 4
---

1 bunch of watercress, trimmed

100 g/4 oz button mushrooms, thinly sliced

50 g/2 oz stoned (pitted) black olives

12 cherry tomatoes, halved

1 quantity of Minted Yoghurt Dressing (see page 183)

1 Separate the watercress into small sprigs. Arrange on four individual plates.

2 Scatter the mushrooms, olives and tomatoes over.

3 Thin the dressing with a little water, if necessary, to give a pouring consistency. Drizzle over the salads.

Tomato and Onion Salad

SERVES 4

4–6 tomatoes, sliced

1 red onion, finely chopped

30 ml/2 tbsp chopped fresh parsley

30 ml/2 tbsp olive oil

15 ml/1 tbsp red wine vinegar

5 ml/1 tsp clear honey

Salt and freshly ground black pepper

1 Arrange the tomatoes overlapping in a shallow dish. Sprinkle with the onion and parsley.

2 Whisk the oil, vinegar, honey and a little salt and pepper together and pour over the salad. Leave to stand for 15 minutes, if time allows, for the flavours to develop.

Chicory, Orange and Cashew Nut Salad

SERVES 4

2 heads of chicory (Belgian endive)

2 oranges

A few fresh coriander (cilantro) leaves, torn

50 g/2 oz/½ cup cashew nuts

1 quantity of Poppy Seed Dressing (see page 184)

1 Cut a cone-shaped core out of the base of each head of chicory and discard.

2 Cut the heads into three pieces and separate into leaves. Place in a salad bowl.

3 Cut all the rind and pith off the oranges, cut the fruit into slices and halve or quarter the slices, depending on size. Add to the bowl with the coriander leaves and nuts.

4 Add the dressing, toss and serve.

Carrot, Courgette and Yellow Pepper Salad

SERVES 4

1 large carrot, coarsely grated

1 large courgette (zucchini), coarsely grated

1 yellow (bell) pepper, coarsely grated

Salt and freshly ground black pepper

45 ml/3 tbsp sunflower oil

15 ml/1 tbsp black mustard seeds

15 ml/1 tbsp sesame seeds

15 ml/1 tbsp lemon juice

1 Put the prepared vegetables in a salad bowl, season with a little salt and pepper and toss gently.

2 Heat the oil in a large frying pan (skillet). Add the seeds and heat gently until they pop.

3 Stir in the lemon juice, pour over the salad and toss gently before serving.

Quinoa Tabbouleh

SERVES 4

100 g/4 oz/1 cup quinoa, rinsed

750 ml/1¼ pts/3 cups water

2 tomatoes, chopped

5 cm/2 in piece of cucumber, finely chopped

1 garlic clove, crushed

5 ml/1 tsp dried mint

30 ml/2 tbsp olive oil

15 ml/1 tbsp lemon juice

Salt and freshly ground black pepper

15 ml/1 tbsp chopped fresh parsley, plus extra for garnishing

1 Simmer the quinoa in the water for about 20 minutes until tender and the liquid is absorbed. Leave to cool.

2 Add all the remaining ingredients and toss well.

3 Leave to stand for 30 minutes, if time allows, for the flavours to develop, then sprinkle with the extra chopped parsley before serving.

Courgette Coleslaw

SERVES 4–6
1 large courgette (zucchini), coarsely grated
½ small white cabbage, coarsely grated
1 large carrot, coarsely grated
1 spring onion (scallion), finely chopped
30 ml/2 tbsp sultanas (golden raisins)
45 ml/3 tbsp Cooked Mayonnaise (see page 181 or buy gluten-free mayonnaise)
15 ml/1 tbsp lemon juice
15 ml/1 tbsp olive oil
5 ml/1 tsp caster (superfine) sugar
Salt and freshly ground black pepper

1 Mix the vegetables and sultanas together in a bowl.
2 Whisk all the remaining ingredients together, seasoning to taste with salt and pepper. Pour over the salad, toss and chill until ready to serve.

Potato and Yoghurt Salad

SERVES 4
450 g/1 lb baby potatoes, scrubbed
30 ml/2 tbsp snipped fresh chives
75 ml/5 tbsp plain yoghurt
30 ml/2 tbsp olive oil
Salt and freshly ground black pepper
Paprika, to garnish

1 Boil the potatoes in salted water until tender. Drain and place in a bowl. Leave until warm but not completely cold.

2 Whisk all the remaining ingredients together, seasoning to taste.

3 Pour over the warm potatoes and toss gently. Sprinkle with paprika and serve warm.

Wild Rice Salad

Wild rice mix is a mixture of long-grain and wild rice (which is actually a grass) and is available from supermarkets.

SERVES 4

175 g/6 oz/¾ cup wild rice mix

100 g/4 oz fresh shelled peas

8 radishes, sliced

100 g/4 oz small button mushrooms, sliced

30 ml/2 tbsp raisins

2 spring onions (scallions), finely chopped

1 quantity of Vinaigrette Dressing (see page 183)

1 Cook the wild rice mix according to the packet directions. Drain, rinse with cold water and drain again.

2 Place in a bowl. Add all the remaining ingredients, toss and serve.

Grilled Sweet Peppers with Olives and Sunflower Seeds

SERVES 4

2 red (bell) peppers, quartered

1 yellow pepper, quartered

1 green pepper, quartered

30–45 ml/2–3 tbsp olive oil

30 ml/2 tbsp stoned (pitted) black olives, sliced

30 ml/2 tbsp sunflower seeds

5 ml/1 tsp coarse sea salt

1 Place the pieces of pepper on foil on a grill (broiler) rack and brush liberally with olive oil until glistening.

2 Grill (broil) for about 6 minutes, turning once until slightly charred and soft.

3 Transfer to a serving platter. Scatter the olives, sunflower seeds and salt over and serve.

Far Eastern Salad

175 g/6 oz/¾ cup basmati rice

10 ml/2 tsp ground turmeric

1 green or under-ripe banana, sliced

15 ml/1 tbsp lemon juice

50 g/2 oz/⅓ cup sultanas (golden raisins)

50 g/2 oz creamed coconut, grated

1 green (bell) pepper, finely chopped

200 g/7 oz/1 small can of sweetcorn (corn), drained

1 green chilli, seeded and finely chopped (optional)

1 fresh mango or peach, peeled and diced, discarding the stone (pit)

30 ml/2 tbsp sunflower oil

Salt and freshly ground black pepper

1 Cook the rice in plenty of boiling, salted water, to which the turmeric has been added, for 10 minutes or until just tender. Drain, rinse with cold water and drain again.

2 Place in a bowl. Toss the banana slices in the lemon juice to prevent browning, then add to the bowl with all the remaining ingredients. Toss well and serve.

VEGETABLE AND SALAD SIDE DISHES   133

DESSERTS

There are plenty of desserts you can enjoy without worrying about their ingredients – all the lovely fruit salads, fresh, soft fruits and cream, compôtes and jellies, to name but a few. But there are other desserts that you thought you would have to miss out on like pies, tarts, crumbles and gateaux. Not any more – just look at the selection in this chapter. Many bought ice-creams are fine, but some may contain gluten, so I have included a few simple ones for you to make, together with versions of some of the most popular puddings I know. Now you can really indulge yourself – and your friends and family!

Apple Crumble

You can, of course, substitute any other fruit in this delicious family pudding.

SERVES 4

450 g/1 lb cooking (tart) apples

30 ml/2 tbsp water

100 g/4 oz/½ cup caster (superfine) sugar

2.5 ml/½ tsp ground cinnamon or cloves (optional)

50 g/2 oz/½ cup rice flour

50 g/2 oz/½ cup potato flour

50 g/2 oz/¼ cup butter or margarine

1 Peel, quarter, core and slice the apples and place in an ovenproof dish with the water. Sprinkle with half the sugar and add the spice, if using.

2 Mix the flours in a bowl. Add the fat and rub in with your fingertips until the mixture resembles breadcrumbs. Stir in the remaining sugar. Sprinkle over the surface and press down lightly.

3 Place on a baking (cookie) sheet and bake in a preheated oven at 190°C/375°F/gas mark 5 for about 45 minutes until golden and the apples are tender. Serve warm.

Mince Pies

Ideally, make the mincemeat at least a week before you want to use it to allow the flavours to develop. Place it in a clean, sealed container and store in a cool, dry place.

MAKES ABOUT 24

100 g/4 oz/1 cup gluten-free shredded (chopped) vegetable suet

1 eating (dessert) apple, grated

450 g/1 lb dried mixed fruit (fruit cake mix)

100 g/4 oz/½ cup demerara sugar

100 g/4 oz/1 cup chopped almonds

Finely grated rind and juice of 1 lemon

2.5 ml/½ tsp ground cinnamon

2.5 ml/½ tsp grated nutmeg

2.5 ml/½ tsp ground mace

1.5 ml/¼ tsp ground cloves

60 ml/4 tbsp brandy, rum or orange juice

1 quantity of Sweet Pastry (see page 175)

Rice flour, for dusting

Sunflower oil, for greasing

Milk or water and caster (superfine) sugar, to glaze

1 Mix together the suet, apple, dried fruit, sugar, almonds, lemon rind and juice, spices and brandy, rum or orange juice. Cover and leave to stand for at least 4 hours (see note above).

2 Cut the pastry (paste) in half. Roll out on a surface dusted with rice flour and cut into rounds, using a 7.5 cm/3 in biscuit (cookie) cutter. Re-knead and roll the trimmings and use a little of the other half of the pastry, if necessary, to make 24 rounds altogether.

3 Roll out the remainder of the pastry and cut slightly smaller rounds for 'lids'.

4 Press the larger rounds into the lightly greased sections of two tartlet tins (patty pans). (Make the mince pies in two batches if you have only one tin.) Fill with mincemeat and top with pastry lids. Brush with milk or water and sprinkle with caster sugar.

5 Bake in a preheated oven at 200°C/400°F/gas mark 6 for about 20 minutes until golden brown. Cool slightly, then remove from the tin and cool on a wire rack.

Jam Tarts

MAKES 12

⅓ quantity of Sweet Pastry (see page 175)

Rice flour, for dusting

45–60 ml/3–4 tbsp jam (conserve) of your choice

1 Roll out the pastry (paste) on a surface dusted with rice flour and cut into 12 rounds using a 7.5 cm/3 in biscuit (cookie) cutter. Place in the sections of a tartlet tin (patty pan).

2 Add a good 5 ml/1 tsp of jam to each tart.

3 Bake in a preheated oven at 190°C/375°F/gas mark 5 for 15–20 minutes until golden brown. Cool slightly, then transfer to a wire rack to cool completely.

Syrup Tartlets

Use the same quantities to make 1 large 20 cm/8 in tart, on a pie plate, if you prefer.

MAKES 12

½ quantity of Sweet Pastry (see page 175)

Rice flour, for dusting

60 ml/4 tbsp gluten-free sponge cake crumbs or breadcrumbs (see pages 169 and 155–7)

60 ml/4 tbsp golden (light corn) syrup

Finely grated rind of ½ lemon

1 Roll out the pastry (paste) on a surface dusted with rice flour and cut into 12 rounds using a 7.5 cm/3 in biscuit (cookie) cutter.

2 Place in the sections of a tartlet tin (patty pan).

3 Spoon the crumbs into each case and top each with a good 5 ml/1 tsp of syrup, then scatter the lemon rind over.

4 Bake in a preheated oven at 190°C/375°F/gas mark 5 for about 20 minutes until golden and bubbling. Remove from the tin and serve warm or cold.

Fresh Raspberry Gâteau

Try using other soft fruit for a change, such as halved strawberries, sliced peaches or nectarines, stoned (pitted) cherries or even bananas, dipped in lemon juice to prevent browning.

SERVES 6

1 Golden Sponge Cake (see page 169)

150 ml/¼ pt/⅔ cup whipping cream

15 ml/1 tbsp icing (confectioners' sugar)

A few drops of vanilla essence (extract)

175 g/6 oz raspberries

30 ml/2 tbsp redcurrant jelly (clear conserve)

15 ml/1 tbsp water

1 Make the sponge and leave to cool, then split in half horizontally.

2 Whip the cream with the sugar and vanilla essence. Place one half of the cake on a serving plate and spread the cut side with the whipped cream, then top with a third of the raspberries, lightly crushed.

3 Top with the second half of the cake. Arrange the remaining raspberries over the top.

4 Melt the redcurrant jelly with the water and brush over the raspberries. Chill until ready to serve.

Christmas Pudding

The pudding can be kept for up to 3 weeks in the fridge after its first steaming.

MAKES ONE 1.2 LITRE/2 PT/5 CUP PUDDING

Sunflower oil, for greasing

50 g/2 oz/½ cup rice flour

50 g/2 oz/½ cup buckwheat flour

5 ml/1 tsp gluten-free baking powder

100 g/4 oz/1 cup gluten-free shredded (chopped) vegetable suet

1 small eating (dessert) apple, grated

100 g/4 oz/⅔ cup raisins

100 g/4 oz/⅔ cup sultanas (golden raisins)

100 g/4 oz/⅔ cup currants

100 g/4 oz/½ cup dark brown sugar

100 g/4 oz/2 cups wheat-free/gluten-free breadcrumbs (see pages 155–7)

2.5 ml/½ tsp ground cinnamon

2.5 ml/½ tsp ground mace

1.5 ml/¼ tsp ground cloves

1 egg

150 ml/¼ pt/⅔ cup pure orange juice

30 ml/2 tbsp rum

---

1 Oil a 1.2 litre/2 pt/5 cup pudding basin and line the base with a circle of greaseproof (waxed) paper.

2 Mix all the dry ingredients well together in a bowl.

3   Beat the egg, orange juice and rum together and add to the mixture. Stir well until thoroughly combined.

4   Turn into the prepared basin and level the surface. Cover with a double thickness of greased greaseproof paper with a pleat in the middle to allow for rising. Twist and fold under the rim to secure.

5   Steam for 4 hours. Re-cover with clean paper, cool, then store in the fridge until ready to use (see note on page 140). Steam for a further 1½ hours before serving.

Plum Clafoutie

SERVES 4–6

350 g/12 oz ripe plums, halved and stoned (pitted)

75 g/3 oz/⅓ cup granulated sugar

250 ml/8 fl oz/1 cup water

Butter or margarine, for greasing

1 quantity of Yorkshire Pudding batter (see page 173)

45 ml/3 tbsp flaked (slivered) almonds

Icing (confectioners') sugar, for dusting

1   Put the plums in a saucepan with the sugar and water. Bring to the boil, reduce the heat and simmer for 6–7 minutes until the plums are just tender but still holding their shape.

2   Grease a 1 litre/1¾ pt/4¼ cup ovenproof dish. Lift the plums out of the saucepan with a draining spoon, reserving the syrup, and arrange in the base.

3   Pour the Yorkshire Pudding batter over and sprinkle with the almonds. Bake in a preheated oven at 220°C/425°F/gas mark 7 for about 30 minutes until golden and cooked through. Dust with sifted icing sugar and serve warm with the plum syrup.

Chocolate Roulade

This makes a lovely Yule Log at Christmas too: simply decorate with a little artificial robin and a sprig of holly. I would not advise you to eat this if you are lactose intolerant.

SERVES 6

175 g/6 oz/1½ cups plain (semi-sweet) chocolate, broken into pieces

4 eggs, separated

150 g/5 oz/⅔ cup caster (superfine) sugar, plus extra for sprinkling

15 ml/1 tbsp hot water

150 ml/¼ pt/⅔ cup whipping cream, whipped

Icing (confectioners') sugar, for dusting

1 Line an 18 × 28 cm/7 × 11 in Swiss roll tin (jelly roll pan) with non-stick baking parchment, so that it comes about 5 cm/2 in above the rim all round.

2 Melt the chocolate in a bowl over a pan of hot water or in the microwave.

3 Whisk the egg yolks and sugar together until thick and pale.

4 Stir in the melted chocolate and hot water.

5 Whisk the egg whites until stiff and fold into the mixture with a metal spoon.

6 Turn into the prepared tin and spread out evenly. Bake in a preheated oven at 180°C/350°F/gas mark 4 for about 15–20 minutes until firm to the touch.

7 Place a sheet of baking parchment on a clean tea towel (dish cloth). Sprinkle with caster sugar. Turn the roulade out on to the paper. Loosen the cooking paper but leave in place. Cover with another clean tea towel and leave until cold.

8 Remove the cooking paper and trim the edges. Spread with the cream. Roll up, using the paper to help. Wrap in the paper and chill until ready to serve.

9 Unwrap and place on a serving plate. Dust with icing sugar and serve cut into slices.

Peach Almond Crisp

Substitute soya yoghurt for crème fraîche if you are lactose intolerant.

SERVES 6

425 g/15 oz/1 large can of sliced peaches in natural juice

1 peach or orange jelly (jello) tablet

300 ml/½ pt/1¼ cups boiling water

150 ml/¼ pt/⅔ cup crème fraîche

25 g/1 oz/2 tbsp butter or margarine

30 ml/2 tbsp golden (light corn) syrup

30 ml/2 tbsp chopped almonds

A few drops of almond essence (extract)

50 g/2 oz/1 cup cornflakes, lightly crushed

1 Purée the peaches and their juice in a blender or food processor.

2 Dissolve the jelly in the boiling water and stir into the fruit purée. Turn into a glass bowl and leave to set.

3 Spread the set fruit jelly with the crème fraîche.

4 Melt the butter or margarine with the syrup in a saucepan. Stir in the nuts, almond essence and cornflakes. Leave to cool slightly, then spoon over the crème fraîche. Leave to cool, then chill before serving.

White Chocolate Snow Gateau

You can also make a dark chocolate version of this moist cake, using plain (semi-sweet) instead of white chocolate. If you are lactose intolerant, you are advised not to eat this.

SERVES 6–8

Sunflower oil, for greasing

175 g/6 oz/1½ cups white chocolate, broken into pieces

3 eggs, separated

175 g/6 oz/¾ cup caster (superfine) sugar

45 ml/3 tbsp warm water

2 egg whites

300 ml/½ pt/1¼ cups crème fraîche

25 g/1 oz/¼ cup plain chocolate, grated, to decorate

---

1 Grease two 20 cm/8 in sandwich tins (pan) and line the bases with greased greaseproof (waxed) paper or non-stick baking parchment.

2 Melt the chocolate in a bowl over a pan of hot water or in the microwave.

3 Put the egg yolks in a bowl with the caster sugar and whisk until thick and pale.

4 Stir the warm water into the melted chocolate and whisk into the sugar mixture.

5 Whisk all the egg whites until stiff and fold into the mixture with a metal spoon. Turn into the prepared tins and level the surfaces. Bake in a preheated oven at 180°C/350°F/gas mark 4 for about 15–20 minutes. Don't worry if the cakes sink slightly in the centre.

6 Remove from the oven, cover with another sheet of baking paper and then a damp tea towel (dish cloth) and leave until cold.

7 Turn out and remove the paper. Sandwich the cakes together with some of the crème fraîche, then pile the rest on top. Sprinkle with the grated plain chocolate and chill until ready to serve.

Pear and Yoghurt Brûlée

SERVES 4

425 g/15 oz/1 large can of pear quarters, drained, reserving the juice

10 ml/2 tsp arrowroot

5 ml/1 tsp lemon juice

2.5 cm/1 in piece of cinnamon stick

150 ml/¼ pt/⅔ cup thick vanilla yoghurt

1 large egg, beaten

45 ml/3 tbsp light brown sugar

1 Chop the pears and place in a 900 ml/1½ pt/3¾ cup ovenproof dish.

2 Blend a little of the pear juice with the arrowroot in a saucepan. Stir in the remaining pear juice, the lemon juice and cinnamon stick.

3 Bring to the boil and cook, stirring, until thickened and clear. Remove the cinnamon and pour over the pears.

4 Whisk the yoghurt and egg together and spoon over. Bake in a preheated oven at 180°C/350°F/gas mark 4 for about 20 minutes until set.

5 Sprinkle liberally with the sugar and place under a hot grill (broiler) until the sugar melts. Serve hot.

Bakewell Tart

For this recipe, use almond instead of vanilla essence (extract) when making the Golden Sponge Cake (see page 169).

SERVES 6

½ quantity of Sweet Pastry (see page 175)

45–60 ml/3–4 tbsp raspberry jam (conserve)

1 quantity of Golden Sponge Cake mixture (see above)

60 ml/4 tbsp icing (confectioners') sugar

A little lemon juice

Glacé (candied) cherries, halved, to decorate

1 Roll out the pastry (paste) and use to line a 20 cm/8 in flan dish (pie pan), on a baking (cookie) sheet.

2 Spread the base with the jam.

3 Make up the Golden Sponge Cake mixture.

4 Spread over the jam and bake in a preheated oven at 180°C/350°F/gas mark 4 for 30–40 minutes until golden brown, cooked through and the centre springs back when lightly pressed.

5 Leave to cool, then mix the icing sugar with a little lemon juice to a thick, creamy consistency. Spread over the sponge and decorate with glacé cherries.

Strawberry Pavlova

*Ring the changes with any soft fruits of your choice
– I particularly like a mixture of orange segments
and blueberries.*

SERVES 8

4 egg whites

225 g/8 oz/1 cup caster (superfine) sugar

15 ml/1 tbsp cornflour (cornstarch)

1.5 ml/¼ tsp vanilla essence (extract)

10 ml/2 tsp white wine vinegar

150 ml/¼ pt/⅔ cup whipped cream, whipped

175 g/6 oz strawberries, sliced

Small sprigs of mint, to decorate

1 Whisk the egg whites until stiff.

2 Gradually whisk in the sugar.

3 Whisk in the cornflour, vanilla essence and vinegar.

4 Line a baking (cookie) sheet with non-stick baking parchment. Spoon the meringue into a 20 cm/8 in round on the sheet, making a slight hollow in the centre.

5 Bake in a preheated oven at 140°C/275°F/gas mark 1 for 1½ hours until a pale biscuit colour, crisp on the outside and fluffy in the centre. Turn off the oven and leave to cool in the oven (this should prevent cracking).

6 Carefully transfer to a serving plate. Fill the centre with whipped cream and top with the strawberries. Decorate with small sprigs of mint and serve.

Crêpes Suzette

SERVES 4–5

1 quantity of Brittany Pancakes (see page 174)

25 g/1 oz/2 tbsp butter or margarine

45 ml/3 tbsp light brown sugar

Finely grated rind and juice of 1 large orange

Finely grated rind and juice of 1 small lemon

45 ml/3 tbsp brandy

1 Make the pancakes.

2 Melt the butter or margarine in a large frying pan (skillet), add the sugar and stir until it melts.

3 Stir in the fruit rinds and juices and simmer, stirring, for 2–3 minutes until the caramel dissolves and a smooth sauce is formed.

4 Fold the pancakes into quarters and place one at a time into the sauce, spooning the sauce over and pushing each one to the side of the pan before adding the next.

5 Pour over the brandy, ignite and shake the pan gently until the flames subside. Serve straight away.

Vanilla Yoghurt Ice Cream

If you are lactose intolerant, you could use all soya yoghurt instead of vanilla yoghurt and crème fraîche, but the result will not be as creamy.

SERVES 6–8

4 eggs, separated

175 g/6 oz/¾ cup caster (superfine) sugar

300 ml/½ pt/1¼ cups thick vanilla yoghurt

300 ml/½ pt/1¼ cups crème fraîche

2.5 ml/½ tsp vanilla essence

1 Whisk the egg yolks and sugar in a bowl over a pan of gently simmering water until thick and pale.

2 Remove from the pan and continue whisking until cold.

3 Fold in all the remaining ingredients except the egg whites. Turn into a freezerproof container and freeze for 2 hours.

4 Turn into a bowl. Whisk thoroughly with a fork to break up the ice crystals.

5 Whisk the egg whites until stiff and fold in with metal spoon. Return to the container and freeze until firm.

Lemon Sorbet

For Orange Sorbet, use oranges instead of lemons and pure orange juice instead of bottled lemon juice. Sharpen with a little extra lemon juice, if liked.

SERVES 8

---

600 ml/1 pt/2½ cups water

225 g/8 oz/1 cup granulated sugar

Thinly pared rind and juice of 2 large lemons

Bottled lemon juice

2 egg whites

---

1 Put the water and sugar in a saucepan and heat gently, stirring all the time, until dissolved. Bring to the boil, reduce the heat and simmer gently, without stirring, for 10 minutes until thickened but not coloured.

2 Add the lemon rind and leave until cold.

3 Make the lemon juice up to 450 ml/¾ pt/2 cups with bottled lemon juice. Add to the syrup. Strain into a freezerproof container.

4 Freeze for 1½ hours until frozen round the edges. Whisk thoroughly with a fork to break up the ice crystals. Freeze for a further 1 hour and whisk again.

5 Whisk the egg whites until stiff and fold in with a metal spoon. Freeze until firm.

Zabaglione with Fresh Pineapple

You can serve the zabaglione without the pineapple, if you prefer.

SERVES 6

1 fresh pineapple

3 eggs

40 g/1½ oz/3 tbsp caster (superfine) sugar

65 ml/5 tbsp medium or sweet sherry

12 angelica 'leaves', to decorate

1 Slice off the green top of the pineapple and cut a slice off the base, then cut off all the rind.

2 Cut the fruit into small chunks, discarding any hard core. Divide the fruit and any juice between six large wine goblets or sundae glasses.

3 Put the eggs, sugar and sherry in a bowl over a pan of hot water. Whisk with an electric mixer until thick, foamy and voluminous.

4 Spoon over the fruit and decorate with the angelica leaves. Serve straight away.

Strawberry and Raspberry Summer Pudding

SERVES 6

1 Golden Sponge Cake (see page 169)

350 g/12 oz strawberries, halved or quartered

350 g/12 oz raspberries

100 g/4 oz/½ cup light brown sugar

45 ml/3 tbsp orange juice

Crème fraîche, to serve (optional)

1 Make the Golden Sponge Cake and leave to cool. Split in half horizontally, then cut each half into six wedges.

2 Use the wedges, cut sides out, to line a 900 ml/1½ pt/ 3¾ cup pudding basin, so that there are no gaps.

3 Put the fruit in a saucepan with the sugar and orange juice. Heat gently, stirring lightly, until the juices run. The fruit should still hold its shape.

4 Spoon the fruit and juice into the sponge-lined basin and top with the remaining sponge pieces. Stand the basin on a plate.

5 Lay a saucer on top, curved side down, and weigh down with heavy weights or cans of food.

6 Chill overnight. The juices should have soaked through the sponges completely.

7 Loosen the edges with a round-bladed knife, turn out on to a serving dish and serve with crème fraîche, if liked.

Refreshing Rhubarb Fool

SERVES 4

---

350 g/12 oz rhubarb, cut into small pieces

25 g/1 oz/2 tbsp butter or margarine

75 g/3 oz/⅓ cup granulated sugar

Finely grated rind and juice of ½ orange

2 eggs, beaten

150 ml/¼ pt/⅔ cup thick plain yoghurt

20 ml/4 tsp strawberry jam (conserve)

1 Put the rhubarb, butter or margarine, sugar and orange rind and juice in a saucepan. Cover and cook gently, stirring occasionally, for about 10 minutes until pulpy. Beat well.

2 Stir in the beaten eggs and cook, stirring, until thick but do not allow to boil.

3 Remove from the heat and leave to cool. Beat in the yoghurt.

4 Turn into four glass dishes. Top each with a spoonful of strawberry jam and chill until ready to serve.

BREADS, BISCUITS AND CAKES

Practically every bread, biscuit or cake sold in shops has some wheat flour in it. And unfortunately, when making your own, you can't just substitute another flour and expect the same results, because it's the gluten in wheat that gives the baked goods their distinctive texture and flavour.

You can buy gluten-free bakes but they tend to be very expensive and, on the whole, taste disappointing. However, the good news is that there is a wheat-free/gluten-free flour available in all good supermarkets. It is more expensive than ordinary flour but makes a passable alternative for general cooking purposes. It clearly states that it is not recommended for yeast cookery but, with a lot of trial and error, I've succeeded in creating a great loaf with it (see page 155). Also in this section, you'll find a super yeast bread recipe using rice flour (see page 156) and a delicious Buckwheat Soda Bread (see page 157). I've also developed a whole range of delicious bakes for you to enjoy – and I do mean enjoy, not just tolerate!

Crusty White Bread

Grate the skin of the apple as well as the flesh: the pectin, which helps the bread to rise, is just under it.

MAKES 1 SMALL LOAF

A little sunflower oil, for greasing

225 g/8 oz/2 cups wheat-free/gluten-free flour, plus a little for dusting

1 sachet of easy-blend dried yeast

2.5 ml/½ tsp salt

1 eating (dessert) apple

15 ml/1 tbsp sunflower oil

200 ml/7 fl oz/scant 1 cup hand-hot water

1 Grease a 450 g/1 lb loaf tin (pan) and dust with a little of the flour.

2 Put all the ingredients except the water in a large mixing bowl and mix well.

3 Add the water and beat well until the mixture forms a thick batter.

4 Turn into the prepared tin. Leave in a warm place to prove for 15 minutes until the mixture almost reaches the top of the tin.

5 Stand the tin in a roasting tin containing about 2.5 cm/1 in boiling water. Bake towards the top of a preheated oven at 200°C/400°F/gas mark 6 for 1 hour.

6 Turn out of the tin, place upside down on the oven shelf and bake for a further 15 minutes to crisp the crust. Cool on a wire rack.

Milk Loaf

A little sunflower oil, for greasing

175 g/6 oz rice flour, plus a little for dusting

2.5 ml/½ tsp salt

15 ml/1 tbsp caster (superfine) sugar

1 sachet of easy-blend dried yeast

15 ml/1 tbsp sunflower oil

1 egg, beaten

150 ml/¼ pt/⅔ cup hand-hot milk

1 Grease a 450 g/1 lb loaf tin (pan) and dust with a little rice flour.

2 Mix the rice flour, salt, sugar and yeast in a large bowl.

3 Add the oil, egg and milk and beat to form a thick batter.

4 Turn into the prepared tin and place in a warm place for 20 minutes until the mixture almost reaches the top of the tin.

5 Place in a roasting tin containing 2.5 cm/1 in boiling water. Bake in a preheated oven at 200°C/400°F/gas mark 6 for 20 minutes. Turn out of the tin, place upside down on the oven shelf and cook for 10 minutes to crisp the crust. Cool on a wire rack.

Buckwheat Soda Bread

MAKES 1 SMALL LOAF

A little sunflower oil, for greasing

100 g/4 oz/1 cup buckwheat flour, plus a little for dusting

100 g/4 oz/1 cup rice flour

5 ml/1 tsp bicarbonate of soda (baking soda)

5 ml/1 tsp cream of tartar

5 ml/1 tsp caster (superfine) sugar

2.5 ml/½ tsp salt

15 g/½ oz/1 tbsp butter or margarine

300 ml/½ pt/1¼ cups milk

1 Grease a 450 g/1 lb loaf tin (pan) or 15 cm/6 in deep, round cake tin. Dust with a little buckwheat flour.

2 Mix the flours with the bicarbonate of soda, cream of tartar, sugar and salt. Rub in the butter or margarine.

3 Mix with the milk and beat well to form a thick batter.

4 Pour into the prepared tin. Bake in a preheated oven at 200°C/400°F/gas mark 6 for 30–40 minutes until risen and browned and the base sounds hollow when the loaf is tipped out and tapped.

Banana Bread

A little sunflower oil, for greasing

2 very ripe large bananas

10 ml/2 tsp bicarbonate of soda (baking soda)

100 g/4 oz/½ cup caster (superfine) sugar

50 g/2 oz/¼ cup butter or margarine, softened, plus extra for spreading

1 egg, beaten

275 g/10 oz/2½ cups rice flour

5 ml/1 tsp ground cinnamon

60 ml/4 tbsp hot water

50 g/2 oz/⅓ cup raisins

1 Grease and line a 900 g/2 lb loaf tin (pan) with greased greaseproof (waxed) paper.

2 Place the bananas and bicarbonate of soda in a food processor and blend until smooth. Alternatively, mash thoroughly in a large bowl.

3 Beat in the sugar and butter or margarine until blended.

4 Add the egg and beat again.

5 Fold in the flour and cinnamon, then add the hot water and the raisins.

6 Turn into the prepared loaf tin and level the surface. Bake in a preheated oven at 180°C/350°F/gas mark 4 for 1¼ hours until the loaf is well risen and a deep golden brown and a skewer comes out clean when inserted down through the centre.

7 Leave to cool slightly, then turn out on to a wire rack, remove the paper and leave to cool. Serve sliced and buttered.

Sesame Crackers

*Ring the changes by adding poppy, caraway or fennel seeds
instead of sesame seeds.*

MAKES ABOUT 15

100 g/4 oz/1 cup buckwheat flour

50 g/2 oz/½ cup rice flour

50 g/2 oz/½ cup potato flour, plus extra for dusting

A good pinch of salt

5 ml/1 tsp cream of tartar

2.5 ml/½ tsp bicarbonate of soda (baking soda)

150 g/5 oz/⅔ cup butter or margarine

30 ml/2 tbsp sesame seeds

90 ml/6 tbsp cold water

1 Mix the flours, salt, cream of tartar and bicarbonate of soda together in a bowl.

2 Add the fat, cut into small pieces, and rub in with your fingertips until the mixture resembles breadcrumbs.

3 Stir in the sesame seeds, then mix with the cold water to form a soft but not too sticky dough.

4 Knead gently on a surface dusted with potato flour. Roll out thinly and cut into about 15 squares or other shapes. Transfer to a baking (cookie) sheet. Prick decoratively with a fork.

5 Bake above the centre of a preheated oven at 180°C/ 350°F/gas mark 4 for about 25 minutes until crisp.

6 Transfer to a wire rack to cool. Store in an airtight container.

Rich Chocolate Brownies

If you are lactose intolerant, I do not advise you to eat these.

MAKES 15

A little sunflower oil, for greasing

75 g/3 oz/¾ cup rice flour

15 ml/1 tbsp cocoa (unsweetened chocolate) powder

2.5 ml/½ tsp gluten-free baking powder

1.5 ml/¼ tsp salt

100 g/4 oz/½ cup granulated sugar

25 g/1 oz/2 tbsp butter or margarine

30 ml/2 tbsp water

100 g/4 oz/1 cup good-quality plain (semi-sweet) chocolate, chopped

5 ml/1 tsp vanilla essence (extract)

2 large eggs, beaten

1   Grease and line an 18 × 28 cm/7 × 11 in shallow baking tin (pan) with greased greaseproof (waxed) paper or non-stick baking parchment.

2   Sift the flour, cocoa, baking powder and salt together in a bowl.

3   Heat the sugar, butter or margarine and water together until the fat melts. Stir in the chocolate and vanilla.

4   Pour into the flour mixture with the eggs and beat well.

5   Turn into the prepared tin. Bake in a preheated oven at 180°C/350°F/gas mark 4 for about 20 minutes or until the mixture is firm to the touch.

6   Leave to cool in the tin, then cut into squares.

Millet Flapjacks

If you are on a wheat-free diet, try substituting rolled oats for the millet.

A little sunflower oil, for greasing

65 g/2½ oz/scant ⅓ cup butter or margarine

30 ml/2 tbsp granulated sugar

15 ml/1 tbsp golden (light corn) syrup

100 g/4 oz/1 cup millet flakes

45 ml/3 tbsp wheat-free/gluten-free flour

1 Lightly grease an 18 cm/7 in non-stick sandwich tin (pan).

2 Melt the butter or margarine, sugar and syrup in a saucepan.

3 Stir in the millet flakes and flour.

4 Press firmly into the prepared tin.

5 Bake in a preheated oven at 180°C/350°F/gas mark 4 for about 20–25 minutes until golden brown.

6 Leave to cool slightly, then mark into wedges with a knife. When completely cold, cut into wedges before removing from the tin.

No-bake Muesli and Ginger Fingers

MAKES 10–15

50 g/2 oz/¼ cup light brown sugar

30 ml/2 tbsp golden (light corn) syrup

75 g/3 oz/⅓ cup butter or hard margarine

350 g/12 oz/3 cups gluten-free muesli (buy ready-made or see page 27)

10 ml/2 tsp ground ginger

A little sunflower oil, for greasing

1 Melt the sugar, syrup and butter or margarine in a saucepan.

2 Stir in the muesli and ginger.

3 Press into an oiled, 20 cm/8 in square, shallow baking tin (pan).

4 Leave to cool, then chill until firm. Cut into fingers and store in an airtight container.

Vanilla Fork Cookies

You can also use this recipe to make Almond Fork Cookies: use almond instead of vanilla essence (extract) and top each cookie with a blanched almond instead of a cherry. Or, for Chocolate Fork Cookies, substitute cocoa (unsweetened chocolate) powder for half the rice flour, and top them with walnuts.

MAKES ABOUT 20

A little sunflower oil, for greasing

50 g/2 oz/½ cup rice flour

50 g/2 oz/½ cup soya flour

2.5 ml/½ tsp gluten-free baking powder

5 ml/1 tsp vanilla essence

75 g/3 oz/⅓ cup butter or margarine, softened

10 glacé (candied) cherries, halved

1 Lightly grease a baking (cookie) sheet with oil.

2 Sift the flours together with the baking powder in a bowl.

3 Add the vanilla essence and butter or margarine and work with a fork until the mixture is blended, then draw together into a ball with your hands.

4 Shape into 20 small balls and place, well apart, on the prepared baking sheet.

5 Dip a fork in water, then use to flatten each ball of dough.

6 Bake for about 15–20 minutes in a preheated oven at 180°C/350°F/gas mark 4 until golden brown.

7 Remove from the oven and quickly press half a glacé cherry on top of each cookie. Leave to cool for 10 minutes, then transfer to a wire rack to cool completely.

Almond Macaroons

For a change, make Hazelnut Macaroons by using ground and whole hazelnuts (filberts) instead of almonds, and vanilla instead of almond essence (extract).

MAKES 10

---

1 egg white

75 g/3 oz/¾ cup ground almonds

75 g/3 oz/⅓ cup caster (superfine) sugar

15 ml/1 tbsp ground rice

1.5 ml/¼ tsp almond essence

10 whole blanched almonds

---

1 Line a non-stick baking (cookie) sheet with gluten-free rice paper.

2 Whisk the egg white until softly peaking but not stiff.

3 Beat in the ground nuts, sugar, ground rice and almond essence.

4 Spoon 10 mounds on to the rice paper, well apart. Top each with a whole nut.

5 Bake in a preheated oven at 160°C/325°F/gas mark 3 for about 25 minutes until pale golden. Remove from the oven and leave to cool.

6 Cut round each macaroon with scissors. Store in an airtight container.

Florentines

If you are lactose intolerant, omit the chocolate.

MAKES 12
50 g/2 oz/¼ cup butter or margarine
50 g/2 oz/¼ cup caster (superfine) sugar
50 g/2 oz/⅓ cup chopped almonds
3 glacé (candied) cherries, chopped
15 ml/1 tbsp angelica, chopped
15 ml/1 tbsp chopped mixed (candied) peel
15 ml/1 tbsp sultanas (golden raisins)
10 ml/2 tsp single (light) cream
100 g/4 oz/1 cup plain (semi-sweet) chocolate

1 Put the butter or margarine and caster sugar in a saucepan and bring to the boil, stirring.

2 Remove from the heat and stir in all the remaining ingredients except the chocolate. Mix well.

3 Put spoonfuls of the mixture, well apart, on two baking (cookie) sheets, lined with non-stick baking parchment.

4 Bake in a preheated oven at 180°C/350°F/gas mark 4 for about 7 minutes or until golden brown. Cool slightly, then transfer to a wire rack to cool completely.

5 Melt the chocolate in a bowl over a pan of hot water or heat briefly in the microwave.

6 Spoon a little chocolate on the underside of each Florentine in turn, spreading to cover the base and leave, chocolate-sides up, to set.

No-bake Cherry and Date Cookies

Those of you with wheat intolerance can use rolled oats instead of millet if you like.

MAKES ABOUT 12

---

50 g/2 oz/¼ cup butter or margarine

45 ml/3 tbsp golden (light corn) syrup

50 g/2 oz/¼ cup caster (superfine) sugar

100 g/4 oz/2 cups millet flakes

A little sunflower oil, for greasing

50 g/2 oz/½ cup glacé (candied) cherries, chopped

100 g/4 oz/⅔ cup chopped stoned (pitted) dates

1 Melt the butter or margarine, syrup and sugar in a saucepan, stirring.

2 Stir in the millet flakes and spoon half into a greased 18 cm/7 in square baking tin (pan).

3 Mix the cherries and dates together and then scatter over the top. Add the remaining mixture, pressing down well. Chill until firm. Cut into fingers.

Raspberry Chews

MAKES 12

50 g/2 oz/¼ cup butter or margarine

45 ml/3 tbsp seedless raspberry jam (conserve)

50 g/2 oz pink marshmallows

100 g/4 oz/2 cups cornflakes, crushed

A few extra marshmallows, finely snipped, to decorate

1 Melt the butter or margarine with the jam and marshmallows in a saucepan, stirring.

2 Stir in the cornflakes and spoon into paper cake cases (cupcake papers). Sprinkle with chopped marshmallows. Chill until firm.

Chocolate Raisin Crackles

MAKES 12

50 g/2 oz/¼ cup butter or margarine

45 ml/3 tbsp golden (light corn) syrup

50 g/2 oz/¼ cup caster (superfine) sugar

30 ml/2 tbsp raisins

30 ml/2 tbsp cocoa (unsweetened chocolate) powder, plus extra for dusting

100 g/4 oz/2 cups cornflakes, crushed

1 Melt the butter or margarine, syrup and sugar in a saucepan, stirring. Stir in the raisins, cocoa and cornflakes.

2 Spoon into paper cake cases (cupcake papers) and chill until firm. Dust with cocoa before serving.

Nutty Nibbles

50 g/2 oz/¼ cup butter or margarine

45 ml/3 tbsp clear honey

50 g/2 oz/¼ cup light brown sugar

60 ml/4 tbsp peanut butter

50 g/2 oz/1 cup crisp puffed-rice cereal

90 ml/6 tbsp chopped mixed nuts

1 Melt the butter or margarine, honey and sugar together in a saucepan, stirring.

2 Stir in the peanut butter, cereal and 15 ml/1 tbsp of the nuts. Chill the mixture until almost firm.

3 Roll into balls and roll in the remaining chopped nuts. Place in paper cake cases (cupcake papers).

Golden Sponge Cake

A little sunflower oil, for greasing

2 eggs

1 egg yolk

65 g/2½ oz/scant ⅓ cup caster (superfine) sugar, plus extra for dusting

1.5 ml/¼ tsp vanilla essence (extract)

40 g/1½ oz/3 tbsp soya flour

40 g/1½ oz/3 tbsp potato flour

40 g/1½ oz/3 tbsp butter or margarine, melted

1 Grease a 15 cm/6 in deep, round cake tin (pan) and line with greased greaseproof (waxed) paper or non-stick baking parchment.

2 Put the eggs, egg yolk, sugar and vanilla essence in a bowl over a pan of hot water and whisk until the mixture is thick and pale and the whisk leaves a trail when lifted out.

3 Sift the flours over the surface and fold in.

4 Add the melted butter or margarine and continue whisking for a further 2–3 minutes.

5 Turn into the prepared tin. Bake in a preheated oven at 160°C/325°F/gas mark 3 for 35–40 minutes until the cake is risen and golden and the centre springs back when lightly pressed.

6 Cool slightly, then turn out on to a wire rack, remove the paper and leave to cool.

7 Dust with caster sugar before serving.

Jam Sponge

Prepare as for Golden Sponge Cake (see page 169) but when cold, split the cake in half horizontally and sandwich together again with about 45 ml/3 tbsp of your favourite jam (conserve).

Butter Cream Sponge

Prepare as for Golden Sponge Cake (see page 169) and split in half horizontally when cold. Make butter cream by beating 50 g/2 oz/¼ cup softened butter or margarine with 100 g/4 oz/⅔ cup sifted icing (confectioners') sugar until smooth. Use to fill the cake and add a layer of jam (conserve), too, if liked.

Chocolate Cream Sponge

Prepare as for Golden Sponge Cake (see page 169) but substitute cocoa (unsweetened chocolate) powder for 15 g/½ oz/2 tbsp of the potato flour. Split the cake horizontally and sandwich together, using a little whipped cream or chocolate butter cream, made by substituting 30 ml/2 tbsp of the icing (confectioners') sugar with cocoa powder in the Butter Cream Sponge recipe above.

Sand Cake

A little sunflower oil, for greasing

A little cornflour (cornstarch) and caster (superfine) sugar, for dusting

100 g/4 oz/½ cup butter or margarine, softened

100 g/4 oz/½ cup caster (superfine) sugar

3 eggs, beaten

175 g/6 oz/1½ cups cornflour

5 ml/1 tsp gluten-free baking powder

Finely grated rind of 1 lemon or orange

A little icing (confectioners') sugar, for dusting

1   Grease a 900 ml/1½ pt/3¾ cup ring mould. Mix a little cornflour and sugar together and use to dust over the surface.

2   Beat the butter or margarine and sugar together until light and fluffy.

3   Beat in the eggs, a little at a time, beating well after each addition.

4   Sift the measured cornflour and the baking powder over the surface and fold in lightly with the lemon or orange rind, using a metal spoon.

5   Turn into the prepared mould and level the surface.

6   Cook in a preheated oven at 180°C/350°F/gas mark 4 for about 1 hour until the cake feels firm to the touch.

7   Cool in the tin (pan) for 10 minutes, then turn out on to a wire rack to cool. Dust with a little sifted icing sugar before serving.

Moist Fruit Cake

This recipe also makes an excellent Rich Christmas Cake. Prepare as below but use dark brown instead of caster (superfine) sugar, double the quantity of fruit and add 15 ml/1 tbsp brandy or rum to the mixture. Bake in a 20 cm/8 in tin (pan) for 1½–1¾ hours.

MAKES A 18 CM/7 IN CAKE

A little sunflower oil, for greasing

175 g/6 oz/¾ cup butter or margarine, softened

175 g/6 oz/¾ cup caster (superfine) sugar

3 large eggs

1 eating (dessert) apple, grated

100 g/4 oz/1 cup soya flour

100 g/4 oz/1 cup rice flour

15 ml/1 tbsp gluten-free baking powder

5 ml/1 tsp ground cinnamon

225 g/8 oz/1⅓ cups dried mixed fruit (fruit cake mix)

150 ml/¼ pt/⅔ cup milk or orange juice (or a mixture of both)

1 Grease and line an 18 cm/7 in deep, round, loose-bottomed cake tin with greased greaseproof (waxed) paper or non-stick baking parchment.

2 Beat the butter or margarine and sugar together until light and fluffy.

3 Beat in the eggs, one at a time.

4 Beat in the grated apple, then sift the flours, baking powder and cinnamon over the surface and fold in.

5 Add the dried fruit and then the liquid to form a soft, dropping consistency.

6 Turn into the prepared tin and level the surface. Bake in a preheated oven at 160°C/325°F/gas mark 3 for 1¼–1½ hours until the top is a rich brown and a skewer inserted in the centre comes out clean. Cover with foil after an hour if over-browning.

7 Leave to cool in the tin for 10 minutes, then turn out on to a wire rack, remove the paper and leave to cool completely.

Yorkshire Puddings

MAKES 12
A little sunflower oil
100 g/4 oz/1 cup wheat-free/gluten-free flour
2.5 ml/½ tsp salt
2 eggs, beaten
150 ml/¼ pt/⅔ cup water
150 ml/¼ pt/⅔ cup milk

1 Pour enough oil to cover the base into each of 12 sections of a tartlet tin (patty pan). Place in a preheated oven at 230°C/450°F/gas mark 8 until sizzling.

2 Meanwhile, put the flour and salt in a bowl. Whisk in the eggs, water and milk to form a smooth, thin batter. Whisk for a further minute.

3 Spoon into the tins and bake near the top of the oven for 20–25 minutes or until risen, golden and crisp on the outside. Remove from the tins and serve piping hot.

Brittany Pancakes

These can be served plain, sprinkled with caster (superfine) sugar and lemon juice, or you can stuff them with any of your favourite fillings – see pages 79 and 148 for two great ideas.

MAKES 8–10

---

100 g/4 oz/1 cup buckwheat flour

1.5 ml/¼ tsp salt

1 egg, beaten

300 ml/½ pt/1¼ cups milk

45 ml/3 tbsp olive oil, plus extra for cooking

---

1 Mix the flour and salt in a bowl.

2 Add the egg and half the milk and beat well. Stir in the remaining milk and the measured oil.

3 Leave to stand for 30 minutes.

4 Heat a little olive oil in a medium frying pan (skillet). Pour off the excess.

5 Add about 30 ml/2 tbsp of the batter and quickly swirl round the pan to coat the base. Cook until holes appear on the surface and the pancake is golden brown underneath.

6 Flip the pancake over and cook the other side briefly until browned. Slide on to a plate and keep warm over a pan of hot water while cooking the remainder. Serve hot.

Savoury Pastry

It's not worth making less than this quantity, even if you don't need it all for a particular recipe. However, it can be kept, wrapped in clingfilm (plastic wrap), in the fridge for 3 days and it freezes well although it becomes a little moist on thawing. Simply knead in a little rice flour until it is no longer sticky before using.

MAKES ABOUT 700 G/1½ LB

450 g/1 lb potatoes, scrubbed and halved or quartered

100 g/4 oz/½ cup butter or margarine

175 g/6 oz/1½ cups rice flour, plus extra for dusting

5 ml/1 tsp salt

1 Cook the potatoes in plenty of boiling water until tender. Drain.

2 Peel off the skins and mash the potatoes well with the butter or margarine.

3 Add the flour and salt and work together to form a dough. Wrap in a plastic bag and chill for 1 hour.

4 Roll out on a surface dusted with rice flour and use as required.

Sweet Pastry

MAKES ABOUT 700 G/1½ LB

Prepare exactly as for Savoury Pastry (above) but use sweet potatoes or yams instead of ordinary ones and omit the salt.

Garlic and Herb Bread Slices

This is a delicious alternative to traditional garlic bread.

SERVES 4

---

25 g/1 oz/2 tbsp butter or margarine

15 ml/1 tbsp olive oil

1–2 large garlic cloves, crushed

15 ml/1 tbsp chopped fresh parsley

2.5 ml/½ tsp dried mixed herbs

Freshly ground black pepper

4 thick slices of wheat-free/gluten-free bread, cut in half diagonally (buy ready-made or see pages 155–7)

---

1 Heat the butter or margarine and oil in a large frying pan (skillet). Add the garlic, herbs and some pepper.

2 Add the bread and turn over in the fat to coat completely. Cook over a gentle heat, turning once during cooking until beginning to brown on both sides. Serve hot.

SAUCES AND ACCOMPANIMENTS

Sauces, dressing and even pickles can be a problem. Here are some delicious versions to enhance all your meals.

Basic Savoury White Sauce

SERVES 4

30 ml/2 tbsp cornflour (cornstarch)

300 ml/½ pt/1¼ cups milk

A good knob of butter or margarine

Salt and freshly ground black pepper

1 Blend the cornflour with a little of the milk in a saucepan and then stir in all the remaining milk.

2 Add the butter or margarine, bring to the boil and cook for 1 minute, stirring all the time until thickened and smooth. Season to taste and use as required.

Cheese Sauce

SERVES 4

1 quantity of Basic Savoury White Sauce (see above)

50 g/2 oz/½ cup Cheddar cheese, grated

Make up the white sauce, then stir in the cheese until melted. Use as required.

Parsley Sauce

SERVES 4

1 quantity of Basic Savoury White Sauce (see above)

30 ml/2 tbsp chopped fresh parsley

Make up the white sauce, then stir in the parsley and use as required.

Béchamel Sauce

300 ml/½ pt/1¼ cups milk

1 bay leaf

1 slice of onion

30 ml/2 tbsp cornflour (cornstarch)

A knob of butter or margarine

Salt and freshly ground black pepper

1 Put the milk in a saucepan with the bay leaf and onion. Bring to the boil, then turn off the heat and leave to infuse until the milk is cold. Strain.

2 Blend the cornflour with a little of the flavoured milk in the rinsed-out saucepan. Stir in the remainder of the milk and add the butter or margarine. Bring to the boil and cook for 1 minute, stirring all the time until thickened and smooth.

3 Season to taste and use as required.

Sweet White Sauce

SERVES 4

---

300 ml/½ pt/1¼ cups milk

30 ml/2 tbsp cornflour (cornstarch)

30 ml/2 tbsp caster (superfine) sugar

A few drops of vanilla essence (extract)

A small knob of butter or margarine

---

1 Blend a little of the milk with the cornflour and sugar in a saucepan. Blend in the remaining milk.

2 Add the vanilla essence and bring to the boil, stirring until thickened, then simmer gently for 1 minute. Stir in the butter or margarine and use as required.

Custard Sauce

SERVES 4

Prepare as for Sweet White Sauce (above) but use 15 ml/ 1 tbsp cornflour (cornstarch) and beat in 2 egg yolks before cooking.

Cooked Mayonnaise

Most recipes use raw eggs, but here is a delicious, cooked version that will keep in a sealed container in the fridge for up to 3 weeks. Use an electric hand beater if possible.

MAKES 150 ML/¼ PT/⅔ CUP

1 egg

20 ml/4 tsp lemon juice or white wine vinegar

150 ml/¼ pt/⅔ cup sunflower oil

Salt and freshly ground black pepper

1 Whisk the egg and 15 ml/1 tbsp of the lemon juice or vinegar in a bowl.

2 Measure the oil in a measuring jug.

3 Place the bowl with the egg in it over a pan of simmering water.

4 Whisk in a little of the oil, then, whisking all the time, continue to add the oil gradually in a very thin trickle, until thick and glossy – about 5 minutes. The mixture should become hot but do not allow to boil or it will curdle.

5 Remove from the heat and whisk in the final 5 ml/1 tsp of lemon juice and a little salt and pepper. Continue to whisk for 1 minute to cool down. Turn into a sealed container, cover, leave until cold, then store in the fridge.

TIP:

You can tell if the mixture does begin to curdle because it will slide away from the sides of the bowl. Remove from the pan of water immediately, whisk in 15 ml/1 tbsp hot water and continue to whisk vigorously for 1 minute.

Aioli

SERVES 4–6

1 quantity of Cooked Mayonnaise (see page 181 or buy gluten-free mayonnaise)

1 large garlic clove, crushed

A good pinch of cayenne

Make the mayonnaise. Whisk in the garlic and cayenne and add a dash more lemon juice, if liked. Use as required.

Tartare Sauce

SERVES 4–6

1 quantity of Cooked Mayonnaise (see page 181 or buy gluten-free mayonnaise)

15 ml/1 tbsp chopped stoned (pitted) green olives

2.5 cm/1 in piece of cucumber, finely chopped

5 ml/1 tsp dried dill (dill weed)

15 ml/1 tbsp chopped fresh parsley

5 ml/1 tsp white wine vinegar

A pinch of caster (superfine) sugar

Mix all the ingredients together. Taste and add a dash more vinegar, if liked. Chill until ready to serve.

Vinaigrette Dressing

SERVES 4

45 ml/3 tbsp olive oil

15 ml/1 tbsp white wine vinegar

1 shallot or very small onion, very finely chopped

15 ml/1 tbsp chopped fresh parsley

5 ml/1 tsp caster (superfine) sugar

A good pinch of salt and freshly ground black pepper

Whisk all the ingredients together and use as required.

Minted Yoghurt Dressing

SERVES 4

60 ml/4 tbsp plain yoghurt

20 ml/1½ tbsp olive oil

10 ml/2 tsp white wine vinegar

5 ml/1 tsp dried mint

Salt and freshly ground black pepper

2.5 ml/½ tsp caster (superfine) sugar

Mix all the ingredients together and use as required.

Poppy Seed Dressing

This is particularly good for dressing salads containing tropical fruits.

SERVES 4–6

60 ml/4 tbsp olive oil

60 ml/4 tbsp red wine vinegar

30 ml/2 tbsp clear honey

10 ml/2 tsp poppy seeds

A good pinch of grated nutmeg

1 shallot, finely chopped

Salt and freshly ground black pepper

Whisk all the ingredients together and use as required.

Dill Pickled Cucumber Slices

SERVES ABOUT 8

½ cucumber

150 ml/¼ pt/⅔ cup white wine vinegar

5 ml/1 tsp dried dill (dill weed)

15 ml/1 tbsp caster (superfine) sugar

6 black peppercorns

1 Cut the cucumber into slices about 3 mm/⅛ in thick. Place in a saucepan.

2 Add the remaining ingredients. Bring to the boil, cover and boil for 1 minute. Leave to cool in the saucepan.

3 Place in a clean screw-topped jar or other sealed container and store in the fridge.

Sweet Chutney

1 very large cooking (tart) apple, cored and quartered

2 onions, quartered

225 g/8 oz/1 cup light brown sugar

225 g/8 oz/1½ cups raisins

225 g/8 oz/1½ cups chopped stoned (pitted) dates

300 ml/½ pt/1¼ cups red wine vinegar

1.5 ml/¼ tsp cayenne

1.5 ml/¼ tsp ground ginger

1.5 ml/¼ tsp ground allspice

Salt and freshly ground black pepper

1 With the machine running, drop the apple and onions into a food processor and finely chop. Alternatively, pass them through a coarse mincer (grinder).

2 Place in a bowl and stir in the remaining ingredients, seasoning to taste with salt and pepper. Cover with clingfilm (plastic wrap) and leave to stand for 24 hours, stirring from time to time.

3 Place in clean screw-topped jars and store in a cool, dark place.

Chilli Salsa

1 red chilli, seeded

3 ripe tomatoes, skinned

200 g/7 oz/1 small can of pimientos, drained

15 ml/1 tbsp tomato purée (paste)

15 ml/1 tbsp red wine vinegar

5 ml/1 tsp light brown sugar

Salt and freshly ground black pepper

Put all the ingredients except the salt and pepper in a blender or food processor and run the machine until smooth. Season to taste. Use as required.

USEFUL ADDRESSES

The Coeliac Society
PO Box 220
High Wycombe
Buckinghamshire
HP11 2HY
01494 437278

The British Allergy Foundation
Deepdene House
30 Bellgrove Road
Welling
Kent
DA16 3PY
Helpline: 020 8303 8583
www.allergyfoundation.com

Action Against Allergy
PO Box 278
Twickenham
TW1 4QQ
020 8892 2711
Please enclose an s.a.e. when writing to the society for information.

The National Society for Research into Allergy
PO Box 45
Hinckley
Leicestershire
LE10 1JY
01455 250715

INDEX

grilled tuna with lentils 106–7

haddock
  spiced haddock kedgeree 32–3
  traditional English fish 'n' chips 121
halibut parcels 105
Halloumi cheese, middle eastern grilled
  supper 85
ham
  baked ham and eggs with cherry
    tomatoes 29
  honey roast ham in cider 94–5
  Parma-style aubergines 54
  pork schnitzels 92
  Westphalian ham and celeriac salad 55
haricot beans, pork and bean
  cassoulet 90–1
hash browns with crispy bacon 34
herring, soused herrings with apple 101
honey nut crunch 23

ice cream, vanilla yoghurt 149
Italian salad with basil and olives 50

jam
  jam sponge 170
  jam tarts 137
  plum barbecued spare ribs 93

kidney, steak, kidney and mushroom
  pie 88–9
kidney beans, chilli con carne with
  crispy tacos 84
kippers and scrambled egg 33

lamb
  chilli con carne with crispy tacos 84
  lamb biryani 80–1
  lamb medallions with rosemary and
    port 77
lasagne al forno, buckwheat 82–3
lemon sorbet 150
lentils, thick red lentil and tomato
  soup 46
lettuce
  smooth lettuce and parsley soup 39
  spiced chicken liver with rocket and
    mango 58
light corn syrup *see* golden (light corn)
  syrup
lima (butter) beans, blushing butter
  beans 126

mackerel in millet 100
mango
  far eastern salad 133
  spiced chicken livers with rocket and
    mango 58
  tropical smoothie 28
marshmallows, raspberry chews 167
mayonnaise
  aioli 182
  cooked 181
  tartare sauce 182
meat
  home-made burgers 64–5
  see also specific meats; minced meat

Mediterranean fish chowder 44
melon and cashew nut cups 52
middle eastern grilled supper 85
milk loaf 156
millet
  honey nut crunch 23
  mackerel in millet 100
  millet couscous with garlic
    chicken 70–1
  millet flapjacks 161
  no-bake cherry and date cookies 166
  spiced muesli 27
mince pies 136–7
minced meat
  buckwheat lasagne al forno 82–3
  chilli con carne with crispy tacos 84
  Polish stuffed cabbage 86–7
minted lemon-glazed chicken 74
minted yoghurt dressing 183
moist fruit cake 172–3
Mozzarella cheese
  Italian salad with basil and olives 50
  pork schnitzels 92
  potato pan pizza 60–1
muesli
  no-bake muesli and ginger fingers 162
  spiced muesli 27
muffins, breakfast 21
mushrooms
  creamy scallops with oyster
    mushrooms 56–7
  cresmolto salad 126–7
  mushroom and artichoke pilau 115
  mushroom and basil tartlets 62–3
  sausages with tomatoes and
    mushrooms 30–1
  seafood pie with mushrooms 97
  spiced haddock kedgeree 32–3
  steak, kidney and mushroom
    pie 88–9
  the great English breakfast 35
mussels, paella 102–3
mustard seed potatoes 124

nasi goreng 87
no-bake cherry and date cookies 166
no-bake muesli and ginger fingers 162
nuts
  almond macaroons 164
  chicory orange and cashew nut
    salad 128
  florentines 165
  honey nut crunch 23
  melon and cashew nut cups 168
  nutty cheese cod 108
  nutty nibbles 168

olives
  cresmolto salad 126–7
  Italian salad with basil and olives 50
onion
  onion bhajis 61
  tortilla 63
oranges
  chicory, orange and cashew nut
    salad 128
  sand cake 171